Ketogenic Diet and Intermittent Fasting Guidebook

Discover the Easy Method That Men, Women, and Even Beginners Are Using for Weight Loss With These Simple Metabolic Therapies in 2019

Leanne Williams Liz Vogel

© **Copyright 2019 - All rights reserved.**

The content contained within this book may not be reproduced, duplicated, or transmitted without direct written permission from the author or the publisher.

Under no circumstances will any blame or legal responsibility be held against the publisher, or author, for any damages, reparation, or monetary loss due to the information contained within this book. Either directly or indirectly.

Legal Notice:

This book is copyright protected. This book is only for personal use. You cannot amend, distribute, sell, use, quote or paraphrase any part, or the content within this book, without the consent of the author or publisher.

Disclaimer Notice:

Please note that the information contained within this document is for educational and entertainment purposes only. All effort has been executed to present accurate, up to date, and reliable, complete information. No warranties of any kind are declared or implied. Readers acknowledge that the author is not engaging in the rendering of legal, financial, medical, or professional advice. The content within this book derived from various sources. Please consult a licensed professional before attempting any techniques outlined in this book.

By reading this document, the reader agrees that under no circumstances is the author responsible for any losses, direct or indirect, which are incurred as a result of the use of the information contained within this document, including, but not limited to, — errors, omissions, or inaccuracies.

Table of Contents

Introduction

Chapter 1: What is Ketogenic Dieting?
- History of Keto Diet
- An Outline for the Keto Diet
- A One-Week Keto Menu

Chapter 2: Side Effects of Ketogenic Diets
- The Keto "Flu"
- Getting Rid of the Keto Flu
- Know the Risk of Yo-Yo Dieting
- Good Fats vs. Bad Fats: All You Should Know
- Bad Fats
- Good Fats

Chapter 3: Effective Tips for Successful Keto Dieting
- Low Carb Is Everything
- Focus on What's Right
- Eat Keto-Friendly Foods
- Engage in Physical Activities
- Eat More Healthy Fats
- Test Ketone Levels
- Track Your Macros
- Change Your Food Environment

Chapter 4: Keto-Friendly Foods

- Proteins
- Fats and Oils
- Fruits and Vegetables
- Dairy Products
- Nuts and Seeds
- Water and Other Beverages
- Spices, Seasonings, and Condiments

Chapter 5: Favorite Keto-Friendly Meals

- Breakfast
- Lunch
- Dinner

Chapter 6: Intermittent Fasting

- How Intermittent Fasting Works for Weight Loss
- Science Behind Intermittent Fasting
- Effects of Intermittent Fasting on Cells and Hormones
- Methods of Intermittent Fasting
- Exercising During Intermittent Fasting
- Tips for Combining Intermittent Fasting with Exercise

Chapter 7: Benefits of Intermittent Fasting

- Weight Loss
- Type 2 Diabetes Risk Reduction
- Brain Health
- Longevity

- Inflammation Reduction
- Immune Regulation
- Insulin Sensitivity Enhancement
- Intermittent Fasting and Chronic Diseases

Chapter 8: Intermittent Fasting in Men vs. Women

- Intermittent Fasting Modifications for Women
- Eat Healthy Fats
- Choose Low-Impact Foods
- Reduce Fasting Period

Chapter 9: Intermittent Fasting and Ketogenic Diet

- Tips for a Successful Keto and Fasting Plan
- Tips on Getting Comfortable With Intermittent Fasting
- Some Avoidable Mistakes

Conclusion

References

Introduction

In many circumstances, you might think that it is entirely acceptable to be considered short, too tall, or even slim. Anything is better than being called fat. Your weight should be watched closely instead of being ignored. For this reason, it has become imperative for everyone to be aware of their diets and to live a healthy life. Aside from the gross disadvantages that come with being overweight as far as physical activities, it also poses adverse health conditions (e.g., heart disease and type 2 diabetes) that may lead to long term issues or death if not properly managed. These issues have led experts to come up with many weight-loss therapy ideas over the years.

Of all the treatments that people have attempted in their journey to be able to lose weight, the ketogenic diet has proven to be very useful when it comes to providing results. Besides its weight-loss benefits, there are numerous other health advantages attached to this therapy. These are the reasons why many doctors have been recommending it to their patients. What's even more impressive is the fact that this treatment, combined with another weight-loss method, known as intermittent fasting, can have more significant results.

In this eBook, will give you a rundown of everything that you will need to know about ketogenic dieting. You will find great ways to lose extra pounds, but more importantly, there are also tips on how to combine this technique with intermittent fasting. At the end of your journey, you are armed with the best ways to proceed with keto dieting and intermittent fasting, understand the dos and don'ts of these weight-loss methods and that you have started seeing positive results that will last.

Thank you and I hope you enjoy this audiobook, the only thing I ask is if you could please leave a review after listening...

Chapter 1: What is Ketogenic Dieting?

The word 'ketogenic' originated from 'ketones,' from which 'keto' is derived. Ketones are a small fuel molecule used as an alternative to providing sugar in the body when glucose (blood sugar) is short in supply. When you are low on carbs, your body goes through a metabolic state known as ketosis. Ketosis is characterized by a rise in the level of ketones in the system. Here you start burning glucose due to the lack of energy. Keto diets, unlike other low-carb diets, are centered on this macronutrient which supplies about 90% of the body's calories. Ketones are created from fats, and they provide energy to the whole body, particularly to the brain. The brain is the powerhouse of the human body, and it is always working. Even when you are asleep. However, it cannot run directly on fat, unless it gets converted into either glucose or ketones.

Whenever there is a drop in the level of insulin in your body, the amount of fat that your system burns spikes because the stored fats become more accessible and make it easier for your body to utilize them. It is a fact that burning fat is one of the easiest ways to shed a few pounds. This process is also beneficial for the body, in the sense that it gives you enough energy and reduces the number of times that you get hungry and helps you stay alert and focused throughout the day. When you are on a keto diet, your body begins to run on fat all day long, so it is perfect for getting your weight under your control since it burns fats 24/7.

Once you have decided to go on a keto diet, you should avoid too much protein because it can easily interfere with ketosis. That's why you need to employ some tricks, as well as a conscious effort, to get the results you desire. For instance, you must eat very low levels of carbohydrates in a day. Keep in mind that there are foods with extremely high levels of carbs, e.g., banana. There are about 27 grams of carbs in a medium sized banana. When you start on a keto diet, you should also remember that reaching ketosis does not take place overnight. Retraining your liver to produce ketones is not an easy feat. It typically takes a few days to get to this metabolic state.

In summary, the keto diet is a low-carbohydrate diet, which is used to burn fat more easily and quickly by allowing you to consume more fats than carbohydrates. It follows a dietary plan of about 60 to 70% fat, 15 to 30% protein, and 5 to 10% carbs (Perfect Keto, n.d.).

Generally, it is considered to be safe for almost everybody, but there are some groups of people to whom special consideration should be given. Those on medication for diabetes or hypertension, as well as mothers that are breastfeeding, should consult with their doctor before starting any diet or lifestyle changes.

History of Keto Diet

Fasting dates as far back as the twentieth century when ancient Greek physicians utilized it as a treatment for diseases like epilepsy and other health issues (Occhipinti, 2018). They also considered it an essential component of a healthy lifestyle. Ketogenic dieting is an eating pattern that birthed in the form of fasting to treat epilepsy in France in the year 1911. For over 2000 years this method has served as a standard practice across the world and is said to be the only treatment for epileptic patients that was recorded by Hippocrates. This is the first known use of the therapy before it was adopted to help people lose weight, which is now its most common use in the contemporary world.

According to a study, patients with epilepsy who took meals with low calories and tried fasting suffered from fewer seizures and less effect from the condition (Occhipinti, 2018). At first, the results from this routine were impressive, but as time passed, it was discovered that they were only temporary since the seizures returned in many patients as soon as they went back to their original diets. This led to doctors focusing their research on eliminating starch and sugars instead of placing an equal restriction on all calories. A particular point of reference is the case of Dr. Wilder of Mayo Clinic, (Occhipinti, 2018) who discovered that patients had fewer seizures when they ate high-fat and low-carb diets.

He created the ketogenic diet as a way of replicating the metabolism that would occur when fasting. Adopting this method kept the patients' bodies in a fasted state by requiring it to burn fat instead of glucose. This convinced the metabolic actions of the body to act as if it was starving, even though it was taking in enough calories and nutrition to sustain it and remain in a comfortable state. A few years later, this therapy became known as the standard keto diet, thanks to Dr. Peterman, another physician of the Mayo Clinic (D'Andrea Meira et al., 2019). In this approach, the fat-to-protein ratio is 4:1. There is a 90% distribution of calories from fat, 6% from protein, and just 4% from carbs. Even though this ratio is considered the standard, 3:1 is also beneficial. His proportions are still used today.

While fasting was useful for the treatment of epilepsy, the keto diet was found to be more sustainable with the same results as fasting (Land, 2018). Since this therapy has now run into its second century, the basic eating strategy has remained relatively unchanged. According to nutritionists, one gram of protein per kilogram of body weight should be consumed, while ten to fifteen grams of carbs should be taken daily (Patz, 2017). The rest should be filled with fat. Initially, doctors placed more emphasis on accurate measurements of foods for better results. Foods were weighed at the time before consumption to ensure that participants were kept on track.

In the 1990s, keto diets became unpopular as they merely served as objects of historical study rather than medical facts (Occhipinti, 2018). It, however, made a comeback in the year 1994, thanks to the TV show called Dateline. In a particular episode in October, a two-year-old boy named Charlie had a case of uncontrollable seizures until he was placed on the keto diet. On the show, viewers saw how the diet reduced Charlie's seizures, and this sparked an outbreak of interest and more scientific research about the method.

After it resurfaced, the keto diet was adopted as a viable option to treat epilepsy once again. It has also gained widespread acceptance and is now available at almost all children's hospitals. People show scientific interest in addition to the role that it plays in neurological disorders.

It is important to note; however, that a keto diet is not only good for just epilepsy. If it were, it would have been less famous since epilepsy isn't a common condition. The most typical use of the diet is for losing weight. Though it is not entirely clear when this diet has become accepted as a weight-loss medium, it is known that the early and late 90s has been dominated by the Atkins diet which shares the same perspective on carbs as the ketogenic diet. The renewed interest on the method made researchers pry into the possible effects that it can have on healthy humans, and the results are quite impressive. Today the keto diet has gained recognition that goes far beyond the mere treatment of epilepsy.

An Outline for the Keto Diet

There is no standard ratio for the measurement of the intake of essential nutrients (carbohydrate, protein, and fat) while someone is on a keto diet, but it sets the drastic cut in the consumption of carbs as its premise. Typically, the advisable ratio for your daily level of carbs should be reduced to 50 grams, which is less than the number of carbs found in a bagel. For better results, you can decrease it further to as low as 20 grams in a day. For a diet of 2000 calories, it is advisable for your meal plan to consist of 165 grams of fat, 75 grams of protein, and 40 grams of carbohydrates. While the level of protein in a keto diet is kept at a minimum ratio, it still provides enough nutrients to preserve body mass, as well as the muscle without preventing ketosis.

Although there are different versions of the ketogenic diet, the carbohydrate consumption is always kept at a minimum while the foods that are high in saturated fats get pushed to the forefront.

Here are the different diets to choose from.

Standard Ketogenic Diet

This diet consists of foods with high fat, moderate protein, and low carbs. The usual ratio is 75% fat, 20% protein, and 5% carbohydrate.

Clinical Ketogenic Diet

When you go through clinical keto dieting, you can expect intervals of high carb refills. This means that you have a few days while on the ketogenic diet and then take a break to consume a high amount of carbohydrates. For example, you decide to go on a five-day keto diet. Right after those five days, plan for a day when you will only eat a lot of starchy foods.

Targeted Ketogenic Diet

Here, when on a keto diet, you are allowed to add carbs around workouts.

High-Protein Ketogenic Diet

This version is similar to the standard keto diet, in the sense that you have to eat more protein than what is recommended. So if you consume 65% fat and 5% carbohydrate, you need 35% protein.

Nevertheless, you should take note that scientists have only been able to gather enough research on the standard ketogenic diet. Both the clinical and targeted keto diets are more often used by bodybuilders and athletes who need to keep their body in peak condition. For this reason, the focus will be more on a standard ketogenic diet in this eBook.

When on a ketogenic diet, it should be followed

faithfully until you shed your desired amount of weight. After that, it is vital to keep up with your weight-loss goal by preventing yourself from gaining extra pounds. To ensure that you keep it off, you are expected to follow the diet for a few days or weeks per month.

The decision to switch to a ketogenic diet may seem overwhelming and complicated. It really doesn't have to, as long as you stick to the dos and don'ts. Reaching a state of ketosis is your primary goal. This is attained by eating a low intake of carbs, so remember that this can only be achieved when the body is deprived of starchy sources. While some individuals may get into a state of ketosis by cutting their carbohydrate level down to 20 grams, others may achieve the same result with a far higher amount of carb consumption. Generally, the lower the intake of carbs, the easier it is to reach and stay on ketosis. This is why it matters to eat keto-friendly foods, such as eggs, chicken, condiments, fatty fish, meat, full-fat dairy, full-fat cheese, nuts and seeds, nut butter, avocado, and other non-fatty vegetables.

The main foods to avoid are pastries (bread and other baked foods), sweets and sugary foods, sweetened beverages beans and legumes, pasta, grains, and grain products (e.g., wheat, rice, oats, and cereals). Starchy vegetables, high-carb sources, fruits, and some alcoholic drinks should also be avoided. Though it is essential to stay away from foods that provide carbohydrates, low-glycemic fruits like berries can be consumed in small amounts as long as you make sure that you are taking them in a macronutrient range. It also is essential to say no to processed foods and unhealthy fats such as margarine, shortening oils, and vegetable oils while sticking to good sources. The examples of processed foods that should be avoided include hot dogs, frozen meals, and fast food. Diet versions of foods that contain artificial colors, sweeteners, and alcohol should be avoided as well.

A One-Week Keto Menu

Just like any other new venture, you may find it quite challenging to come up with a perfect menu for your keto diet. Remember, even though this can be uncertain, it does not have to be complicated. The first thing to keep in mind when planning your meals is that everything you consume has to have more fat and fewer carbs. So, here is an example of a simple yet perfect menu for your one-week keto diet.

Sunday

Breakfast: Coconut milk chia pudding with coconut and walnuts on top.

Lunch: Cheese and turkey, avocado Cobb salad made with greens and hard-boiled eggs.

Dinner: Coconut chicken curry.

Monday

Breakfast: Two eggs with pasteurized butter and sautéed green vegetables.

Lunch: Bunless grass-fed burger with cheese, avocado, and mushrooms on top a bed of greens.

Dinner: Pork chops with green beans sautéed in coconut oil.

Tuesday

Breakfast: Mushroom Omelet.

Lunch: Tomato stuffed with tuna salad on top of a bed of greens with celery on the side.

Dinner: Grilled salmon with spinach sautéed in coconut oil.

Wednesday

Breakfast: Bell pepper stuffed with egg and cheese.

Lunch: Arugula salad with hard-boiled eggs, avocado, turkey, and blue cheese.

Dinner: Roast chicken in cream sauce with sautéed broccoli.

Thursday

Breakfast: Keto granola toppings on full-fat yogurt.

Lunch: Cauliflower rice steak bowl with cheese, salsa, herbs, and avocado.

Dinner: Bison steak with cheesy broccoli.

Friday

Breakfast: Baked avocado egg boats.

Lunch: Caesar salad with chicken.

Dinner: Pork chops with vegetables.

Saturday

Breakfast: Cauliflower toast with cheese and avocado toppings.

Lunch: Bunless salmon burgers with Pesto toppings.

Dinner: Zucchini noodles and meatballs with parmesan cheese.

As you can see in the above menu you can have different and nicely flavored meals, even when you are following a keto diet. Though most of these foods are based on animal products, the menu is also beneficial for vegetarians as there is a wide range of vegetables to choose from here. Recipes for all of these items can be found on the internet.

You may want to consider snack options from the extensive list of keto-friendly snacks available out there as well. Keep in mind that snacking between meals can help you keep hunger at bay and help you to stay on track.

Chapter 2: Side Effects of Ketogenic Diets

As mentioned earlier, even though the science behind it has not been proven yet, the keto diet has been a very potent remedy for cases of seizures in children with epilepsy. Francine Blinten, a certified nutritionist and public health consultant, who has used the diet on cancer patients with peculiar conditions, warns that the keto diet will do more harm than good, especially in people with kidney problems.

While there are a whole lot of gains such as weight loss and other health benefits when you go the ketogenic way, some experts frown at the diet, stating that there are more risks associated with a high level of fat (BMJ, 2016). According to a few of them, the diet is a total no-no when it comes to using it to lose weight due to the not-so-pleasant side effects that may occur with it. As well as its unsustainable nature. Other professionals who are in favor of the diet also agree that, if it isn't executed well, it might become disastrous to you while following the diet. So, if you intend to choose the keto technique to shed a few pounds, you may want to study the possible downsides that are connected to it.

The ketogenic diet is gradually taking precedence over all other weight-loss therapies. People across the globe who want to lose weight have embraced it as a way of burning fat in as few as ten days. Though the proponents of this diet say that it is an easy way to make the body burn its own fat through low-carb dieting and that it provides more energy to dieters, nutritional experts claim that it is not a safe method to lose body fat. While others believe that it is an easy way to enter starvation mode as the body merely loses water weight while on a keto diet. According to them, when the body enters into ketosis, it begins to lose muscle, leading you into a fatigued state, then eventually extreme hunger. Some folks refuse to back up this idea, but they say that they do not recommend the diet to someone who wants to gain muscle. The heart, after all, is also a muscle and is at risk when you subject yourself to a keto diet. This points to the fact that the weight-loss technique cannot be entirely safe for the muscles. Therefore, it is more advisable to try the ketogenic diet under the supervision of a clinical expert instead of doing it on your own for an extended period.

Here are some symptoms that going on a ketogenic diet can cause and you should consider before starting on this journey.

The Keto "Flu"

The keto flu is a combination of several physical indications that begin to manifest in someone who follows a ketogenic diet. While it is comprised of different symptoms, it feels like influenza. This is the result of the adaptation of the body to a new diet that consists of a little number of carbohydrates. As you may recall that in the keto diet, the body is forced to produce ketones, which are the byproducts of fat. Because of that, they replace glucose and become the primary source of energy. In normal circumstances, ketones are kept in reserve to provide power when simple sugar is not available. The switch takes place in rare cases of starvation or fasting. When the body begins to be deprived of carbohydrates during keto dieting, it reaches a state of ketosis. That is the time when the diet starts working. Due to this, you may not feel too well at first. This is when you might begin to suffer from the keto flu. The symptoms of this condition come in the form of vomiting, constipation, nausea, and irritability. You will also begin to urinate continually due to the high level of ketones produced by the body during the breaking down of fat. These ketones then get flushed out of your system through frequent and increased urination. The high rate of urination also leads to the uncontrollable loss of electrolytes, which then aggravates these symptoms. You will then be dehydrated and experience other indications of influenza, including dizziness, fatigue, and muscle soreness. The fact that carbohydrates are the significant sources of energy and stimulations makes you, who is short of it, crave sugar, experience brain fog, and have difficulty concentrating. It is similar to the signs of withdrawal.

Though the flu-like symptoms can range from mild to severe, they also vary from one to another. The signs typically start to manifest within the first few days of the diet and may last for about one week. In some people, though, the indications remain longer. They can also become causes of grief. Even to the extent that some dieters may use it as a sufficient reason to give up. The good news, however, is that there are ways to reduce the symptoms of keto flu. It is also important to note that the flu is not contagious, so there should absolutely be no cause for alarm.

Getting Rid of the Keto Flu

The symptoms of the ketogenic flu can stress you out since it may last for a week or more. You may also find it extremely challenging to adapt to the diet, but here are a few tips to help your system go through the transition phase more quickly.

Hydrate Yourself

For your general well-being, it is vital to stay hydrated. When you are trying to adopt the keto diet, you may want to consider drinking more water than you are used to, to allow your body to accept the new routine faster and reduce the symptoms of keto flu. When you try this diet, you shed water more efficiently. The reason for this is that glycogen, which is the stored form of carbohydrates, binds with water in the body. The glycogen levels are forced to drop with the reduction of dietary carbohydrates. Thus causing water to be excreted from the system. Hydration will help reduce symptoms like fatigue and muscle cramping. For this reason, it is imperative to replace fluids when you are experiencing diarrhea in association with keto flu since it can also cause an additional loss of bodily fluids.

Replace Electrolytes

If you are trying to tackle the keto flu, it is crucial to replace dietary electrolytes by getting adequate amounts of minerals that provide them.

Insulin is an essential hormone that absorbs glucose from the bloodstream. During the keto diet, the level of insulin decreases, causing the kidneys to release an excess quantity of sodium from the body. There are a lot of dietary restrictions that come with the ketogenic diet, especially when it comes to foods that are high in potassium, such as beans, fruits, and starchy vegetables. When your goal is to adopt this diet, you need to make up for these nutrients to be able to push through the entire journey. To acquire minerals, you should look for foods that are capable of maintaining a healthy balance of electrolytes. These can be avocados, leafy vegetables, and of course, salt. Not to mention higher levels of magnesium can help to reduce muscle cramps, headaches, and sleep issues.

Get Enough Sleep

In the early phase of the ketogenic diet, fatigue and irritability seem to be some of the major complaints that you might hear among individuals who are attempting to adapt to this regimen. The keto flu can worsen due to lack of sleep because it causes an increase in cortisol. Cortisol is a stress hormone that is released by the adrenal glands that affect your mood. If you are experiencing the keto flu, and are finding it difficult to sleep, here are some tips that may help:

1. Cut out ambient lights

When trying to doze off, lights are the most significant distractions. Luckily, it is easy to deliberately block them out by staying away from anything and everything that produces light. Draw the blinds, shut off your mobile phone, television, and computer in your bedroom to create a favorable environment for restful sleep.

2. Take a bath

Just before you get ready to go to sleep, make sure you relax your nerves and muscles by taking a shower or a bath. They are an effective way of calming every part of your body and feel refreshed. It is also a good idea to add Epsom salt or lavender oil to your bath water to help your system to wind down and relax as you prepare for bedtime.

3. Reduce your intake of caffeine

Not only is it a known fact that caffeinated drinks are addictive, but it is also important to note that they may affect your sleep by keeping you awake for longer hours than you typically want to. You should train yourself to stay away from caffeine in the early stages of the ketogenic diet or when you are suffering from the keto flu. If you must drink caffeinated beverages, make sure that you have them early in the day when you do not need to go to sleep. A good rule is to not have anything caffeinated after mid-day. This will guarantee that, by evening, you are finally ready to take that much-needed rest since the drink has undoubtedly worn off by that time.

4. Create a stable sleeping pattern and wake up early

It is easy for your body to get used to a particular routine if you have subjected yourself to it over a specific period. Following one specific sleeping and waking pattern will help your system shut down and wake up at times based on how you have programmed it to. This way, your sleep pattern will normalize, and you can boost the quality of your rest.

Stick to Less Strenuous Exercises

While exercises are absolutely beneficial for weight loss and overall well-being, it is also essential to stay away from activities that are capable of straining your muscles and the rest of your body. This is an especially useful tip for individuals who are experiencing the keto flu. Some of the symptoms that are common in the first week of the diet are stomach discomfort, fatigue, and muscle cramps. These are only a few reasons why you need to give an adequate amount of rest to your body during this phase. Even though activities like cycling, weightlifting, running, and other strenuous workouts may seem like a go-to when you are on your weight-loss journey, it is essential to shelve these exercises for the time being. You need to allow your system enough time to adapt to its new fuel sources. You can still exercise, but it is a better option to participate in activities such as yoga, leisure biking, and walking.

Eat Enough Fats and Transition Slowly

When introducing the keto diet to your body, it's essential to keep in mind that you will not be able to adopt the entire program all of a sudden. It is a good idea to take it slow. The first stage of the diet may force you to crave foods that are not part of the ketogenic plan, e.g., bread, pasta, bagels, and cookies. Seeing fat as the primary source of energy will reduce your cravings and give you a sense of satisfaction over time. If you have a hard time getting rid of carbohydrates, you should gradually eliminate them instead of staying away from them all at once. As you get rid of carbs little by little, you should substitute them with fat and protein to allow your body to have a smooth transition and decrease the symptoms of keto flu in the process.

Reduce the Risk of Kidney and Heart Damage

When on a ketogenic diet, you may be prone to acute kidney damage as a result of the loss of electrolytes such as potassium, magnesium, and sodium. This is caused by constant urination, which has the potential to lead to dehydration, lightheadedness, kidney injury, or kidney stones. Someone who follows this program can also be at risk of developing cardiac arrhythmia. The minerals that are lost when you urinate are essential to keep the heart beating regularly. Electrolyte deficiency can be detrimental to your health as it may result in irregular heartbeat, which may prove to be fatal.

According to research in the Journal of Child Neurology, 13 out of the 195 epileptic children who were placed on the keto diet developed kidney stones (Kim, 2017). It was, further noted, however, that those kids who were given potassium citrate were less prone to kidney stones than the others. For these reasons, experts have advised that those who wish to go with this dietary plan should speak to their healthcare practitioner if they have kidney-related concerns. If a man consumes a lot of meat (mainly processed ones when on a diet), for instance, he will be more susceptible to kidney stones and gout. Gout is a severe and excruciating metabolic disease that causes high levels of uric acid in the blood and joints, causing pain. After all, while a high intake of animal protein increases your calcium and uric acid levels, the combination of kidney stones and high uric acid cannot keep you away from gout. Generally, the ketogenic diet is not so friendly with people who have kidney diseases. In truth, they are usually placed on a strict, low-protein diet by their doctors. This regulation may not align with the low-carb, high-protein pattern that keto dieters may need to follow.

While the ketogenic diet relies on a high level of fat to burn calories, it is essential to know that certain types of fat are not healthy to some parts of the body. For instance, saturated fats and your heart are not friendly with each other. To maintain a healthy heart, you have to stay clear of foods like butter, cheese, and red meat. When shopping for groceries, you should try to read the labels so that you know if they contain ingredients that might bring you more chaos than calm health-wise. Things like hydrogenated oils (a.k.a. Trans fat) should be avoided as they are capable of increasing the low-density lipoproteins (LDL), which are commonly known as "bad" cholesterol in the body while reducing the high-density lipoproteins (HDL) or "good" cholesterol. According to the American Heart Association (n.d.), such fatty acids will heighten your chance of heart diseases and stroke probability. These issues should be taken into consideration when deciding on the quality of fats that you will consume. If you want to try the keto diet, you ought to eat more plant-based unsaturated fats, which have been proven to protect the heart. E.g., olive oil, avocado oil, nuts, and seeds. If your system is already high in cholesterol, you should consult your doctor before starting to follow this diet to avoid putting your well-being at a higher risk.

It is essential to note that experts have contrasting views on the subject of cardiovascular health while on the ketogenic diet. While some researches show that the program may decrease the possibility of having heart disease, as well as the number of saturated fats, others claim that it increases the cholesterol and triglyceride levels of the keto dieters.

Know the Risk of Yo-Yo Dieting

Even though ketogenic dieting began as a treatment for children who were suffering from epilepsy, it has now gained widespread acceptance among adults who are hoping to lose weight. Its fast-growing popularity is connected to the fact that the diet helps people shed a few pounds in as little as one month. According to a research in the American Journal of Clinical Nutrition, obese men who tried the modified version of the keto diet, which involved eating more protein and less carbohydrates, lost about 14 pounds in a month compared to the control group that followed a medium-carb diet and merely lost around 10 pounds (Thorpe, 2017).

The good news is that some professionals say that the individuals who are on the program can keep the weight off entirely if they stay on the diet for a long time. Nonetheless, such a feat is not usually easy to accomplish. When you lose weight during the keto diet, and then you go back to your original eating habits, the reduced pounds are bound to return in no time. Regaining the weight that you have already lost may lead to more negative eating habits. One example of that is called yo-yo dieting, which leads to an increase in abdominal fat accumulation and a higher risk of diabetes. It is essential to stick to a particular diet to achieve long-term success than just the plan itself. For people who have social engagements and are exposed continuously to carb cravings, keto seems to be restrictive and harsh. It becomes increasingly difficult for them to follow the diet for the long term. Once they begin to see positive results, they ditch the program and return to their regular routine. When you turn to yo-yo dieting, you start to hang between the advantages and disadvantages of losing and gaining weight. Hence, yo-yo dieting is also known as weight circling, and it becomes almost inevitable.

Simply put, yo-yo dieting is the pattern of losing weight, regaining the weight that was lost, and losing it again. It is risky, in the sense that it leads to an increased appetite, which can cause you to gain extra pounds over time. It can also lead to a high percentage of body fats and muscle loss. Fatty liver, diabetes, heart disease, and high blood pressure are some of the risks associated with this habit. Yo-yo dieting may not be as bad as weight gain, but it is certainly not as good as weight loss. While research has yet to prove whether being overweight is worse than this technique or not, it is clear that it is better to make small, beneficial, and permanent changes on your diet to promote a healthy lifestyle. Even if the reduction of fats may be slow, the long-term modifications will improve your life and may also prolong it. And there may be a noticeable improvement in your physical fitness as well.

There are other potential side effects of the keto diet. These can include fatigue, irregular menstrual cycles, constipation, bad breath, sleep issues, and decrease in bone density. Aside from that, the effect on blood cholesterol levels has not been thoroughly studied because of the difficulty of tracking dieters on a long-term basis to discover the lasting results of the dietary plan. Nutritionists are also concerned that the high intake of fats, which are considered unhealthy, can hurt someone's health in the long run. The short-term effect that is manifested by the diet, which comes in the form of weight loss, makes it quite challenging to monitor the data as it can be confusing. When an overweight person loses weight, the heart becomes healthier, and the risk of diabetes decreases. Obese people tend to end up with better blood lipids and glucose levels once they start to lose weight. Another disadvantage of the diet is the fact that it limits the number of certain vegetables, legumes, fruits, and grains, which are often considered "unhealthy" in this program. While folks avoid these foods, they miss out on some essential phytochemicals, fiber, vitamins, and minerals that can only be found in those forms. Nutrient deprivation bears significantly negative health impacts, including the increased potential of acquiring diseases and loss of bone mass. The craving for weight loss, which leads most people to go on keto diets, makes them prone to health deficiencies as well due to the low amount of whole foods that are supposed to keep you from contracting cardiovascular illnesses, Alzheimer's, cancer, osteoporosis, as well as type 2 diabetes. The standing question is: are people willing to risk their well-being for short-term goals such as losing weight?

Good Fats vs. Bad Fats: All You Should Know

When it comes to health and nutrition, fats do not have the same rave reviews that vitamins and other nutrients have that seem to reassure people. This may cause you to feel skeptical about relying on fats to lose weight, considering that it is generally perceived as something to be avoided. The truth is, while some fats are bad for your cardiovascular health and overall well-being, other types can be beneficial, and people are advised to imbibe them as part of their diets. So, instead of staying away from them, it is better to go for the good while ditching the bad. But there is no way to eat essential fats if you have no clue about the differences between the two.

While research on continues to evolve, there are a few facts worth talking about. Dietary fats, also known as fatty acids, are obtained from plants and animals. They have been linked to some not-so-pleasant effects on the heart, while others have been proven to have significant health benefits. Often, people tend to underrate the importance of fats in the body, even though their value is similar to that of proteins and carbohydrates when it comes to giving energy. After all, there are bodily functions that rely on fats. To be specific, some vitamins need them to be able to enter the bloodstream and provide nutrients to the body. If you are entirely devoid of fats, chances are, those vitamins may not be in your system as well. All the same, you should consume fatty sources in moderation because excess calories can make you gain weight. While all foods and oils have fats in them, the more dominant type will determine whether they are good or bad for your body.

Bad Fats

These fatty acids are considered to be harmful to your health as they expose you to more health risks. The two types of bad fats are saturated and trans fats. Most foods that contain such fats stay solid when they are kept at room temperature. Such as beef or pork fat, shortening, and margarine.

Saturated Fats

Saturated fats come from animal products, especially high-fat meats and dairy goods. They can also originate from dark chicken flesh and poultry skin, fatty cuts of meats from beef, pork, and lamb, tropical oils like coconut oil, palm oil, and cocoa butter, lard, as well as dairy foods like whole milk, butter, cheese, sour cream, and ice cream. The term "saturated fat" refers to hydrogen atoms, which surround individual carbon atoms. Fatty acids contain a chain of carbon atoms, binding as many hydrogen atoms as possible. This means that it is saturated with hydrogen.

When a diet is rich in saturated fats, it causes the cholesterol level to shoot up, thus tilting the balance towards a more harmful low-density lipoprotein (LDL) and causing blockages in the arteries and other parts of the body. For this reason, nutritionists advise that saturated fats should be reduced to below 10% of calories in a day (WHO, 2018). The intake of foods that are rich in such fatty acids will, therefore, increase the level of cholesterol and LDL in the blood.

For ages, doctors have blamed the consumption of high cholesterol to heart damage, but the idea is now being questioned by modern healthcare experts. A study conducted by Harvard University researchers (2019) suggests that high levels of cholesterol may not be as bad as they are presumed to be when it comes to maintaining a healthy heart. A meta-analysis of 21 subjects revealed that the evidence that could prove that saturated fats are the causes of heart diseases was not enough (Harvard Health Publishing, 2015). Various researchers have found that cardiovascular health risks can now be reduced by replacing saturated fats with polyunsaturated ones. While the reduction rate may be low, the difference can benefit someone's health superbly. We recommend that the HDL should be compared to your total cholesterol level, as well. When the ratio is high, the experts believe that it is associated with the increased resistance of insulin and heart problems. The research concludes that polyunsaturated fats like vegetable oils and high-fiber carbohydrates are the best ways to reduce the risk of cardiovascular diseases. It is important to note, however, that it is quite dangerous to replace saturated fats with highly processed carbohydrates because the result may be the opposite of what you are looking to accomplish.

Trans Fats

Trans fats cannot be produced naturally; they are industrially made. They are absolutely detrimental to your health, and they must be avoided at all costs. During production, they go through a process that adds hydrogenated vegetable oil to solidify them. These fats make people three times more susceptible to health risks (such as coronary heart disease and stroke) than other fats. The reason is that they increase the LDL cholesterol levels while increasing the HDL cholesterol levels. These fats have also been linked to inflammation of the body, which is also capable of leading to heart diseases, diabetes, and stroke.

Basically, trans fats are not crucial to human life as they do not promote good health in any way. According to the Harvard School of Public Health (2019), about 50,000 cases of fatal heart attacks each year have been associated with trans fat. It is related to an increased risk of developing type 2 diabetes as well. Because food companies find these fats cheap and easy to produce, can be used several times in commercial fryers and they have a long shelf-life and appealing taste, they have become more and more popular. These are a few of the reasons why trans fats are used in fast-food outlets and restaurants.

Some states in the United States have either already banned trans fat or are in the process of doing so. As a result of labeling laws, the manufacturers that make claims of no trans fats or zero grams of trans fat, still have hydrogenated oil content. It is, therefore, essential to read through labels before purchasing certain food products to limit the risks of eating harmful ingredients.

Good Fats

These are the types of fats that are considered to be healthier to consume. "Good" fats refer to either monounsaturated fats or polyunsaturated fats. When placed at room temperature, these fats tend to stay liquid. A straightforward example of these fats is vegetable oil.

Monounsaturated Fats

Monounsaturated fats are those that contain fewer hydrogen atoms compared to saturated fats. If you look at their chemical structure, they also have a bend at the double bond, as well as a single carbon to carbon double bond. It is these components that make it liquid when the oil is kept at room temperature. Canola, olive, peanut, avocado, high-oleic safflower, and sunflower oils are excellent sources of monounsaturated fats.

The discovery of the health benefits of the monounsaturated oil can be traced back to the Steven Countries Studies of the 1960s when it was discovered that those in Greece and other Mediterranean areas were less susceptible to heart diseases even though their diets were high in fats. The dominant fats in their eating plans were not the saturated animal type that was common in countries with high rates of heart disease; instead, the inhabitants mostly used olive oil, which contained monounsaturated fats. This has made the Mediterranean diet and olive oil the objects of interest to many people and is now considered as healthy options. To replace the effects of saturated and trans fats, experts claim that people should eat as much of monounsaturated fats as possible.

Polyunsaturated Fats

Polyunsaturated fats are regarded as essentials fat because the body needs them to function, although they cannot be produced naturally. Such fats contain two or more double bonds in their carbon chains. They have two types as well: the omega-3 and the omega-6 fatty acids. The unique numbers in these names represent the distance between the beginning of the carbon chain and the first double bond. Polyunsaturated fat is primarily sourced from plant-based foods and oils. It is excellent for heart health as it lowers cholesterol levels and decreases the risk of having cardiovascular disease.

Omega-3 fatty acids have proven to be very beneficial to the heart. Aside from guarding your heart against illnesses, it also lowers the blood pressure and prevents irregular heartbeat. Sardines, salmon, herring, and trout are examples of fish that contain omega-3 fatty acid. If you cannot eat fish, you can also find these polyunsaturated fats in walnuts, flaxseed, and canola oil. Omega-6 fatty acid, on the other hand, is present in roasted soybeans and soy nut butter, walnuts, tofu, margarine, pumpkin seeds, sesame seeds, sunflower seeds, corn oil, sunflower oil, sesame oil, and other vegetable oils.

When polyunsaturated fat is eaten in place of highly refined carbohydrates and saturated fat, the harmful LDL cholesterol levels may decrease, and your cholesterol profile may improve. Also, triglycerides are reduced by this type of good fat. Omega-3 fatty acids may be useful in the treatment of strokes as well. Not only do they raise the HDL level, but they also make sure that your heart rhythm will not dangerously rise. There is evidence that points to the fact that polyunsaturated fats reduce the need for corticosteroid medications of people who suffer from rheumatoid arthritis. There is another research (albeit still inconclusive) that states that omega-3 may improve your chances of avoiding dementia as well (Harvard Health Publishing, 2015).

Chapter 3: Effective Tips for Successful Keto Dieting

You may already know the importance of a keto diet to your health; that's why you are determined to start this therapy. Chances are, you also believe that the journey is going to be a smooth one. Well, even though it is not necessarily challenging to achieve ketosis, it will be foolhardy to think that it is going to be a walk in the park. Since you are entirely new to this path, there is no need to act like an expert, you should be focusing on knowing what to do and how to do it right.

Truth is, the ketogenic diet is not as much about what you do but how well you do it. The better you are at adapting to all the twists and turns of this therapy, the higher the probabilities are of achieving success in a short time. This section takes you through some valuable information on how to reach ketosis and find keto dieting success.

Low Carb Is Everything

The most essential element of the ketogenic diet is the absolute reduction of carbohydrate intake. Though this may not sound super-secret, there are some intricacies that you must learn to execute the process well. While the body relies on glucose or sugar as a fuel source, it can also make use of other reserves like fatty acids and ketones. Glucose is stored in the liver in the form of glycogen and can be converted to energy. When there is a low level of carbs, these glycogen stores are depleted. It lowers the level of insulin in the body, thus forcing a release of fatty acids from fat deposits. The liver then transforms these fatty acids into acetone, acetoacetate, and beta-hydroxybutyrate, which can then be used to fuel some parts of the brain.

For different individuals, there are varying levels of carb restrictions needed to induce ketosis, but the Atkins diet recommends consuming 20 grams of carbs daily or less for about two weeks to induce ketosis. Once you have attained ketosis, you can then add little amounts of carbohydrates to your diet, making sure that you continue to maintain this metabolic process (Spritzler, 2016). A previous study carried out in one week showed that the people who were suffering from type 2 diabetes reduced their carb level to less than 21 grams daily and experienced the excretion of ketones through the urinary glands 27 times more than their baseline levels (Spritzler, 2016). Another study, however, allowed adults with type 2 diabetes to eat 20-50 grams of carbs daily, depending on the number of carbs that kept them in ketosis within a target of 0.5 to 3.0 mmol/L (Spritzler 2016). In contrast to these results, if you are following a keto diet for therapeutic purposes, your carbs should be restricted to less than 5% of calories or 15 grams per day to boost ketone levels. You should try the program under the supervision of a healthcare expert only.

Focus on What's Right

There are a lot of theories in the keto dieting world. For someone who seeks answers and hopes to get the diet right, they may be contradictory. The need to find the correct answers to fitness-related questions should take precedence over everything. You do not want to invest all your energy on practicing what you think is the real keto diet, only to find out later that you are doing something else. You ought to understand the proper process to do the ketogenic program. Thus, you must concentrate on important things (such as the consumption of a high amount of fats) instead of doing rigorous exercises. After researching, you will find that the reason why keto dieters lose weight is that they eat fewer calories than they are used to. No matter what the level of restriction you place on carbs may be, you can merely burn your own fat by depriving yourself of calories. Your focus, therefore, should be on looking for a diet plan that will allow you consume fewer calories without dealing with cravings and feeling hungry - a couple of issues associated to the early stage of the keto diet. Once you manage to find that kind of diet, you already have a sustainable way to lose weight.

To create a caloric-deficit diet, you should consider these two principles:

- Eat satiating foods that are rich in protein and fiber.
- Get rid of all processed foods that are always rich in calories since they are easy to binge on.

One of the reasons why the keto diet promotes weight loss fast is that it follows the ideas mentioned above more than other popular diets. This results in the feeling of being sated in people who are following the keto diet, even though they are consuming fewer calories. They begin to burn excess fat, which is the common end-goal of individuals who are in the program. If you have been on the keto diet for a while, and you are not getting the results that you want, perhaps it is time to focus less on carb restriction and start eating fewer calories than your body requires to maintain your weight. Being in a caloric deficit is one of the essential keys to losing weight while on the keto diet, and the best way to achieve this is by eating keto-friendly foods, which will be discussed below.

Eat Keto-Friendly Foods

As you may already know, keto-friendly meals refer to foods that are extremely low in carbs. This low-carb level varies for each person, but it is typically restricted to 20 grams per day. To maintain this benchmark, however, you will have to tackle your cravings while checking every food that you consume. After all, most of the things you eat contain a lot of carbs. It may be surprising to you to discover that some natural foods you tend to love (like a banana) will drag you closer to and even over the caloric benchmark that has been set. Though they are high calories, and sugar seems to be everywhere, you should not feel discouraged as there are equally delicious meals that can help you stay faithful to your low-carb diet. Here is a list of foods that you ought to think about while following the ketogenic plan:

- Lamb, poultry, eggs, fish, and beef
- Low-carb vegetables, such as spinach, broccoli, kale, and cauliflower
- High-fat dairy products like full-fat cream, hard cheese, butter, and so on
- Avocados, blackberries, raspberries, and other low-glycemic berries
- Sweeteners like erythritol, monk fruit, and stevia
- High-fat salad dressing, coconut oil, etc.

Some foods that should be avoided because of their high-carb contents are:

- Wheat, rice, cereals, corn, and other grains
- Apples, oranges, bananas, and other fruits
- Maple syrup, honey, agave, and all other types of sugar
- Potatoes, yams, and other tubers

In addition to the keto-friendly foods listed above, there are baked and fried foods that are made from keto flours that originate from coconut, almond, and similar ingredients. Remember that staying away from carbs does not guarantee weight loss. Even when you eat fewer carbohydrates, if you do not maintain a low-caloric level, you may continue to struggle with weight gain. Hence, it is essential to know how much fats, carbs, and proteins you consume daily.

Engage in Physical Activities

Some studies have shown that people on the keto diet also need to engage in a certain level of physical activities for best results. Ketosis, according to these researches, also help in boosting athleticism. When you are more active, you are likely to reach ketosis faster. During exercise, after all, the level of glycogen in the body plummets and are in turn replenished with the level of carbohydrates, which are then converted to glucose before getting transformed into glycogen once more. When there is a low intake of carbs, there is nothing to replace the glycogen that is expended during exercise, so the liver is forced to produce ketones, which are used in place of glycogen to provide fuel for the muscles.

An investigation states that when the ketone concentration in the blood is low, exercise serves as a booster to the level at which ketones are produced. Besides, the ketone levels may rise as well when one works out in a fasted state.

It is important to note, however, that although exercises boost ketones, it may take a while, about four weeks, for the body to fully adjust in making use of ketones and fatty acids as its primary source of fuel. During this period, it may be a good idea to tone down the physical activities intensity temporarily.

Eat More Healthy Fats

To reach ketosis quickly, it is ideal to consume a lot of healthy fats more regularly. Recall that a low-carb keto diet does not rely on the reduction of carbohydrates alone, but also the increase in fat level. When you are on the keto diet, you draw about 65% to 75% of your calories from fats.

The first step to taking an adequate amount of fat is

knowing that they are not dangerous. The good fats will not expose you to heart disease or make you gain weight as long as they are not eaten with carbohydrates. As already stated in the previous chapter, though, there are bad fats that should be totally avoided to keep them from endangering your well-being.

Test Your Ketone Levels

It is an absolute fact that people's bodies and metabolisms are different. While some can handle stress better, other individuals cannot. While a few find it difficult to sleep, many people fall to sleep, rest, or relax very quickly. Some are more physically active than others, too.

To ensure that you are correctly following the diet, it is essential to test your ketone levels to establish carbohydrate and protein baselines for your personal tolerance. There are a couple of ways to do this, but the most effective is by using a blood ketone meter. With these apparatuses, you will be able to know your blood ketone level by the pricking a tip of your finger, similar to how a glucometer is used to test blood sugar for diabetics. These devices will establish whether or not you are in nutritional ketosis. You can easily find a *Precision Xtra* or *Keto Mojo*. Both are inexpensive and do not require a prescription to purchase at a pharmacy.

Light nutritional ketosis falls between 0.5-1.5 mmol/L. You'll be getting a decent effect on your weight, but it is not yet at a peak level. Around 1.5 – 3 mmol/L is what's called optimal ketosis and is recommended for maximum weight loss. Within the first two weeks of the strict keto diet, most people find their ketosis level within the range of 0.5-3.0 mmol/L since the body has now been deprived of glucose. It is making use of fat and producing ketones as a byproduct. You should test your blood ketone level once a week, switching between mornings and evenings alternatively, to find out if your system is remaining in ketosis. After your body has fully adopted the keto diet from 4 to 6 weeks, you can now gradually introduce some proteins, sweet potatoes, and even berries to your meal plan. After that, you should test your blood ketone level the following morning to know whether or not you are still in ketosis. If you are, it shows that your body is insensitive to insulin enough to handle extra protein and carbs and always enjoy the benefits that come with being in ketosis. All this information will be beside the point if you don't take the test.

Track Your Macros

People tend to underestimate the number of calories they consume daily. There is always a difference between the calories you think you are getting and the calories that you actually consume. You may feel that you have cut down your caloric intake, but you are still not losing weight. In reality, some people still manage to lose weight on some low-calorie days, even though their subconscious weight-regulating mechanisms manage to get more calories the next day. The result is that you will gain more weight or reach an all-time-high weight loss level that may be difficult to recover from. Sadly, many dieters fail to grasp what is really happening. They start to blame themselves or their diets. The truth is that they only need to take some time and evaluate the amount of food that they are eating to know where adjustments should be made and what food items need to be avoided entirely. You can monitor the things that you eat by employing the use of calorie tracking apps and a scale. By combining both tools, you will be able to devise an accurate knowledge of your food choices and lose weight consistently. This will help you to avoid eating more calories than you might consume if you have measured the food beforehand, and you will also be able to know what your caloric and macronutrient needs are.

When buying a scale, you may want to consider the following features:

1. Make sure it has a conversion button.

Most scales with conversion button usually has the ounce-to-gram or gram-to-ounce conversion button. This will make food measurement easier to follow because most calorie-tracking devices use a mixture of units.

2. Look for an automatic shutoff.

Before buying a scale, make sure to find out if the apparatus has an automatic shutoff feature. If it does, it may be difficult for you to measure food if it switches off on its own. To be on the safe side, look for a device that allows you to either program the automatic shutoff or will enable you to turn it off manually.

3. Choose a scale that has a removable plate.

If you measure wet ingredients, it can be challenging to clean the plate if it is not removable. You will need to wash that part of the scale sometimes to be sure that you don't get sick. It is a good idea to buy a scale with a detachable plate for easy cleaning.

4. Look for the tare function.

It is easier to weigh things on scales that allow you to place plates, bowls, or cups on them. With the tare function, the scale reverts to zero when you place an item on top of it.

When you take the time to track the weight of the foods you eat, you can ensure that you will be able to meet your weight-loss goals.

Change Your Food Environment

Your food environment is another crucial factor that impacts what and how much you eat. Even with all the necessary mechanisms in place, it is still possible for you to cheat on your diet. It is even easier when you are traveling, or there is a special occasion. This is why it is of utmost importance to be aware of your food environment.

The food environment is:

The physical presence of food that affects a person's diet,

A person's proximity to food store locations,

The distribution of food stores, food service, and any physical entity by which food may be obtained, or

A connected system that allows access to food (Designed for Disease, 2008).

The food environment is also known as the community food environment, nutritional food environment, or local food environment. The retail food environment includes the community level (e.g., presence and locations of food stores, markets, or both) and the consumer level (e.g., healthful, affordable foods in stores, in markets, or in both) (Designed for Disease, 2008). Your food environment is evolving at a faster pace than ever before. The truth is, our brains and bodies are not wired to handle the abundance of food that has become a staple in our modern food environment. There are increasingly extensive options of dishes to choose from: fast foods to processed foods, organic, and gluten-free. They come in all different forms. For someone who is trying to stay faithful to a diet, it's easy to trigger our desires, because they are always readily available, and your brain pushes you to go for foods that do not require you to work for them. If you choose to act on the signals that your mind sends out, you may find yourself going for calorie-dense foods like french fries, pizza, cakes, cookies, etc. This can cause you to snack in between meals to energize yourself and eating more than you should. This often leads to overeating, which results in weight gain. It is as if we keep reminding ourselves that we need to prepare for famine, even though the famine never comes. It's easier to gather calories and gain weight than lose it. You can prevent these surging desires by giving yourself room to stick to the diet to be able to lose weight.

To achieve this, here are some things you may want to consider:

1. Have meal plans

Planning for the foods you will eat at every meal is an excellent way to stay faithful to your keto diet. Whether you are in transit or just at home, you want to prevent yourself from succumbing to food temptations. When you are on vacation, make sure you have premade meals or keto-friendly snacks. If that is not possible, go to restaurants with keto-friendly options. When at home, prepare meal plans (possibly a meal timetable) that give you all the nutrients that you need and nothing more.

2. Keep only keto-friendly foods around

It may be difficult, but sticking with ketogenic foods is not impossible. When hunger sets in, we may be pushed to act against our own will because, at this point, the only thing the body cares about is how to satisfy your cravings. Whatever rules you may have set for yourself rarely matter when you feel hungry. It makes you vulnerable, and it becomes easy to convince yourself to cheat on your diet.

Planning for the worst is the best option in this case.

Ensure that keto-friendly foods are the ones that are within your reach. If you are struggling with overeating keto-foods, try to keep the foods that need some level of processing before eating. This way, you will end up eating fewer calories since you may feel discouraged to eat when you know you have to unwrap or prepare a lot of things.

3. Stick to foods you can measure and track

If you think that adding extra oil, cheese, and or meat to your meals does not mean anything, you would be wrong. These extras are also capable of adding to your weight. You should stick to your macronutrient goals by eating what is necessary for you. If you do add anything extra to a meal, track it to keep yourself heading in the right direction.

At first glance, greasy foods may not look as if they pose a threat to your diet. The more you add to each meal, however, the more they add up. These can halt your progression or add on the weight that you have been working so hard to lose.

4. Avoid eating convenient foods impulsively

Since some foods are quite natural to munch on, we seem to keep them close at hand. While they may be suitable for satiating hunger, they are just as dangerous to your diet if you do not learn to control your ingestion rate.

The indulgence of tasty and convenient foods should be kept at a bare minimum. When you know that you have a favorite keto-friendly snack or meal, you must monitor how you eat them. Make sure you do not have more than one serving at your disposal at a particular point in time unless you are planning on having that meal for the next day. For every food that you know that you can eat without stopping, make it difficult for yourself to consume more of it than you can.

5. Chose a meal plan that works for you

It is important to note that there is no one-size-fits-all approach to the keto diet. What has worked for your friend or sibling may not work for you. People are all wired differently, and metabolic processes are as unique as fingerprints. When you are starting your keto journey, take note of those meals that work best for you, and stick with them. You will try various plans before deciding which of them the best fit is for you. While you're at it, try not to be so quick to switch programs. Remember that the first phase of the diet can be a bit delicate, and you don't want to make yourself uncomfortable by using yourself as a lab rat. Once you notice that your system is responding positively to a particular meal plan, keep up with it for as long as possible before moving on to another if you ever feel the need to switch.

Enjoying this book so far? I'd love it for you to share your thoughts and post a quick review on Audible!

Chapter 4: Keto-Friendly Foods

Deciding what to eat when on a keto diet may be tricky as your food choices are now limited to stuff with extremely low carbs. The selection problem aside, without having an idea of what keto-friendly options are available, the whole process may be all for nothing since you may find yourself muddying your diet with foods that you are expected to stay away from in the first place.

We have come up with a list of foods that can be associated with the ketogenic process to help you figure out what to buy and what to eat. While sticking to the 5% carbs rule that comes with the diet, here are the groups of foods you can choose from for your keto-friendly meals.

Proteins

A significant factor to note when it comes to proteins is that the higher the amount of protein in a food, the lesser the quantity of that food consumed should be. When you limit your protein intake to pasture-raised and grass-fed options, you minimize the risk of taking in bacteria and steroid hormones that other meat products have. In red meats, there isn't too much to be scared of. Although added sugar, salt, and other processed ingredients are found in cured meats. When buying steaks, consider going for fatter cuts like the rib-eye. Ground beef for hamburgers or other meals, fattier ratios like 85:15 or 80:20 are advised. For poultry, darker meats contain more fat than white varieties, so it is better to stick to them. Whitefishes, on the other hand, are not only rich in protein but also give you Omega-3.

Remember that you do not need too much protein when you are on a keto diet as they lead to lower levels of ketones and an increased level of glucose. With this in mind, when dealing with meat, make sure you are mindful of protein intake. Keep in mind that you are aiming for nutritional ketosis. You can, however, play an easy trick by trying to balance out your proteins and eating fattier side dishes. If you decide to eat lean beef, you will have to be careful with the proportion of protein. Do not forget that jerky and other beef snacks can pile up your protein level fast as well, so make sure to accompany it with a portion of fatty food like cheese.

If you do not eat pork or beef, lamb can be substituted in its place. Cuts of meat like bacon can be replaced with similar leaner items, too. You can add extra fat if you deem it necessary.

To get protein on a ketogenic diet, here are some options to look into:

- Beef: Use steaks with fattier cuts wherever

possible. Roasts, ground beef, stew meats, and steaks are good ideas.
- Poultry: Duck, pheasant, quail, chicken, and any other wild game.
- Fish: Anything caught in the wild like catfish, halibut, mackerel, flounder, mahi-mahi, cod, trout, snapper, tuna, and salmon.
- Shellfish: Oysters, crabs, lobsters, scallops, mussels, squid, and clams.
- Pork: When consuming pork, be on the lookout for added sugars and stick to the fattier cuts. Pork chops, ground pork, ham, pork loin, and tenderloins are a wonderful source of protein.
- Offal/organs: These are very excellent sources of vitamins and other nutrients. They are made up of the internal organs of an animal, including heart, kidney, liver, and tongue.
- Bacon and sausage: Check the labels and watch out for anything cured in sugar or those that have other fillers.
- Whole eggs: If possible, get free range from the local market. There is a variety of ways to prepare them, such as scrambled, poached, fried, boiled, and deviled.
- Nut butter: It is better to go for natural and unsweetened while sticking with the fattier options like almond butter and macadamia butter. Be careful with the consumption of legumes (e.g., peanuts) as they are high in omega-6.
- Other Meats: You should stick to fattier cuts of turkey, veal, lamb, goat, and other wild game.

When you do eat meat, it is fine to have it in moderation. Always remember that the intake of proteins must be in balance with fat.

Fats and Oils

Recall what we have already discussed about good and bad fats in the second chapter. When choosing your foods, it is essential to apply your knowledge regarding their differences by choosing to obtain fats from natural sources like fruits and nuts. You can also use ingredients like butter, coconut oil, olive oil, etc.

When on a ketogenic diet, fats and oils will be the majority of your daily caloric intake. It is crucial to keep the things you like or dislike under consideration while creating your meals. There are several ways to add fats and oils to your meals, either in the form of toppings or dressings. For polyunsaturated and monounsaturated fats, to be specific, foods like egg yolk, coconut oil, olive oil, macadamia, avocado, and nuts are less inflammatory and chemically stable for most people.

It's important to balance your consumption of omega-3 and omega-6 as well; that's why you should go for fish such as tuna, trout, wild salmon, and shellfish. If you are not a fan of seafood (or you are allergic to them), you may choose to take fish oil supplements. Krill oil is also a good source of omega-3. Fruits and nuts, however, can be extremely high in omega-6 so you may want to eat sources like peanuts, pine nuts, walnuts, and almonds in moderation. Safflower and corn oils are also excellent sources of omega-6 as well. To keep your fatty acids at a healthy range, you should not overindulge in desserts that have a high concentration of almond flour. Even though these essential fatty acids provide humans with some core nutrients, they are mostly not balanced in a standard diet.

Here are some fresh ideas for keto-friendly foods that are rich in good fats and oils:

- Coconut butter
- Olive oil
- Cocoa butter
- MCT
- Avocado oil
- Macadamia oil
- Coconut oil
- Olive oil
- Macadamia/Brazil nuts
- Mayonnaise
- Butter/Ghee
- Egg yolks
- Tallow
- Fatty fish
- Avocado
- Lard
- Animal fat (non-hydrogenated)

When you are making use of vegetable oils that come from soybeans, safflower, flax or olive, it is better to go for "cold-pressed" options if they are available. In case you prefer to fry things up, you should choose non-hydrogenated lard, ghee, coconut oil, or beef tallow since these oils have higher smoke points than other types. A higher smoke point means that you will get a greater concentration of essential fatty acids from them.

Fruits and Vegetables

Vegetables are a crucial part of the keto diet, but there are times when we get stuck because of some decisions made and regret them later. Green, leafy vegetables remain the best option when it comes to selecting the right sources for your keto-friendly meals. Some vegetables are very high in sugar and do not contribute positively to our diet, so the decision to cut those out of your diet is vital for the program's success. When following a ketogenic diet, eating vegetables that are high in nutrients and low in carbohydrates are the best options. These can be included in almost every meal as well. They are mostly leafy and dark vegetables - anything that shares semblance with spinach or kale. It is a good idea to go for cruciferous vegetables that are grown above the ground.

Organically grown vegetables are good, as they do not have pesticide residue. Besides the harmful chemicals, though, there is not much difference between the organic and non-organic varieties. As research has shown, their nutritional qualities are the same. This means that there is no need to feel too bothered if you cannot get the organically grown vegetables as the non-organic ones are just as good. Both frozen and fresh options are available year round, so there are not many limitations when it comes to choosing what to eat. If you wish to consume vegetables that have grown below the ground, you should do so in moderation. To be specific, you need to be careful with the number of carbohydrates that they have. Often, underground vegetables are used as flavorings for foods and are very easy to regulate. For example, you can use half an onion for a whole pot of soup.

When choosing your vegetables, you should divvy up your choices according to their carb rate. You should try as much as you can to limit your intake of the following fruits and vegetables:

- High-carb vegetables: garlic, onion, mushroom, parsnip, potatoes, starchy vegetables, and squash
- Citrus: orange, lemon, and lime in both juice and recipes
- Nightshades: eggplant, pepper, and tomatoes
- Fruits: bananas, blackberries, raspberries, strawberries, and blueberries

Some of the most common keto-friendly vegetables are cabbage, cauliflower, broccoli, romaine lettuce, spinach, baby bella mushrooms, green bell pepper, yellow onions, and green beans.

Dairy Products

Milk-based products are mostly keto-friendly, so any type is acceptable. You may, however, want to stick to full-fat dairy items.

Dairy products are consumed with other meals on the keto diet as they are not to be eaten as main dishes, but you should consume them at a minimal level. Typically, most of the meals in this plan come from fats/cooking oils, proteins, and vegetables. When eating dairy products, it is preferable to eat organic choices since the processed ones always have about two to five times higher levels of carbohydrates, and they add up with time. Full-fat dairy products are preferable as opposed to low fat or fat-free products, which have significantly higher levels of carbohydrates. If you are sensitive to lactose, it is better to go for long-aged dairy products because they have less lactose concentration. Examples of dairy items that can be eaten when following a keto diet are:

- Hard cheeses: aged cheddar, parmesan, Swiss, feta, and so on
- Soft cheeses: Brie, Colby, Monterey Jack, blue, and mozzarella
- Spreadable: cream cheese, mascarpone, crème Fraiche, sour cream, etc.
- Heavy whipping cream
- Mayonnaise and mayo alternatives that are also rich in dairy
- Greek yogurt

If you are looking for ways to add extra fat to your meal, you can prepare fatty side dishes or sauces like creamed spinach. Keep in mind; however, they are rich in protein as well, so you have to be careful when pairing them with foods that are already loaded with protein.

It is essential to pay close attention to your body when consuming dairy products. If you have noticed that you have either reached a plateau or slowed down in losing weight, you may have to think about reducing your dairy intake.

Nuts and Seeds

First of all, you should know that peanuts are prohibited in the keto diet because they are legumes. That said, nuts are best consumed when roasted since the process removes harmful nutrients and reduces their level of acidity. Raw nuts are mostly used as flavorings to foods and for adding texture. You can have them for snacks as well. While this may be rewarding, it may be a bad idea for your weight-loss goal since nuts may work against it in the long run. Snacking on nuts generally raises the level of insulin in your body. That's why they may slow down your ability to lose extra pounds. While they are a great source of fats, it is vital to keep in mind that they also have carbohydrates and proteins. Protein in nut flours, in particular, can quickly accumulate; when using them, you have to be aware of the amount that you use. Omega-6 fatty acids are also one of the nutrients found in nuts. Typically, you may want to consider sticking with the fattier options since they happen to have a lower amount of carbohydrates.

Here are things to consider before deciding to open a bag of nuts when you are on a ketogenic diet:

- Brazil nuts, macadamia nuts, and pecans are fatty, low-carb choices. They can be eaten with meals or as fat supplements.
- Hazelnuts, pine nuts, and walnuts contain a moderate amount of carbohydrates. They should be eaten only for texture or flavor.

- Cashews and pistachios are to be avoided or rarely eaten as they have a very high concentration of carbohydrates. Cashews, for instance, has almost as many carbs as you need to survive for an entire day.

Brazil nuts, pecans, macadamia nuts, almonds, and hazelnuts are the most common keto friendly nuts available.

Nuts and seed flours are excellent substitutes for regular flours. In keto, seeds and nuts are often associated with baked desserts. Almond flours and flaxseed meals are standard products used, but it's essential to eat them at a moderate level. You can experiment with your baking recipes by mixing different flours to get a consistent texture that will mimic wheat flour. This mixture will lead to lower carb counts in recipes. You should be aware of the fact that flours react differently. Primarily when used in baking. While coconut flour, for instance, will absorb more water, almond flour will not require as much liquid. These flours are not only useful for baking alone, but you can use them to coat your meat before frying. Also, they can serve as the base for foods like pizza. With enough creativity, you will be able to recreate an old-time favorite by creating a low carb version of it.

Almond flour, coconut flour, chia seed meal, flaxseed meal, unsweetened coconut, etc. are some of the keto-friendly nut/seed items you may consider choosing from.

Water and Other Beverages

For beverages, water is always the best idea. Not only does it keep you healthier, but it is more hydrating than anything else. You may decide to add flavorings to your water by adding lime/lemon juice.

For most people who have started trying the ketogenic diet, dehydration is a widespread side effect that's caused by the natural diuretic effect of the program. If you are prone to bladder pain and urinary tract infections, you are advised to prepare more for this if you wish to go on the keto diet. For the first weeks, prepare yourself to drink at least eight glasses of water daily. This is very important to stay hydrated, so you should drink more water than you are probably used to while following the ketogenic process.

If you can recall, dehydration and the lack of electrolytes are significant causes of keto flu. Considering two-thirds of the human body is made up of water, experts advise that people should stay hydrated all day, regardless of whether you are on the keto diet or not. It depends on your size, weight, activity level, and where you live. In general, you should try to drink between half an ounce and an ounce of water for each pound you weigh, every day. For example, if you weigh 150 pounds, that would be 75 to 150 ounces of water a day. If you live in a hot climate and exercising a lot, you'd be on the higher end of that range; if you're in a colder climate and mostly sedentary, you'd need less. (Nessler, 2009). For many individuals, keto approved beverages and coffee do the trick to up their energy rate and added fats. To help stay hydrated, replace one serving of a caffeinated drink with a glass of water. You will also need to be conscious of the fact that you need to replenish your electrolytes by drinking bone broth or sports drinks that are flavored with sucralose or stevia.

Below are some examples of keto-friendly beverages:

- Water: This is your everyday source of hydration. As one of the building blocks of life, it is easily accessible to you. You may choose to drink either sparkling or regular water.
- Bone broth: This liquid provides electrolytes that can kick start your energy. It is also loaded with nutrients and vitamins.

- Coffee: With some added weight loss benefits, this beverage helps in improving your mental focus.
- Tea: Even though not many people find this enjoyable, it has the same effects as coffee. If you choose to drink tea, try to stick with white or green tea. It has less caffeine than other teas do as well as added weight loss and health benefits.
- Coconut/Almond Milk: This can easily replace your favorite beverage. The unsweetened versions are your best options.
- Flavorings: Those packets that are flavored with sucralose or stevia are the best when it comes to taste. Alternatively, you may add a squeeze of orange, lime, or lemon to your water bottle.
- Alcohol: Try to stay away from beer and wine as much as you can. If you must drink alcohol, go for hard liquor. Nonetheless, remember that too much alcohol will slow down your weight-loss process.

Spices, Seasonings, and Condiments

Spices and seasonings are a fundamental part of everyday cooking. Without them, food would be bland and unenjoyable. Who wants to eat plain chicken? When it comes to the keto diet, though, it can be very tricky. Even though they may come off as small ingredients, they are capable of adding extra carbs to a meal. If you wish to be strict with your seasonings, ultimately you will have to consider staying away from processed foods. Even though there seems to be a lot of low-carb condiments in the market, most of them have a high concentration of glycemic sweeteners, and you may want to avoid them.

When you are tracking your overall carb level, you should add spices to your calculations because they also contain carbohydrates. Often, premade spice mixtures contain sugars, so be sure to go through the nutrition label before consuming them to know what they are. For salt, you can choose sea salts over table salts as they are often powdered with dextrose. If you can, do not add more sugar to your spice blend or foods.

Below are some common keto-friendly spices and seasonings.

- Rosemary
- Oregano
- Cayenne pepper
- Cinnamon
- Cumin
- Basil
- Chili powder
- Parsley
- Thyme
- Cilantro

Consequently, you can add salt and pepper to your food without much worries about their nutritional information.

It will always be better for you on a keto diet to stick to homemade foods than processed ones. The more real food you consume, the more you can control the ingredients that go in it. Even though it is acceptable to consume processed foods, many of them out there are not very good for the keto diet. For this reason, you should check food labels before buying or consuming anything.

Chapter 5: Keto Friendly Meals

If you have come this far with us, then it's safe to say that you are prepared to go head-on into the ketogenic program. The success of your journey largely depends on the food that you eat, as well as the proportions and nutritional values of the foods that you consume. To help you, we have combined a list of keto friendly meals, broken down into breakfast, lunch, and dinner ideas. You will find an extensive variety of food in this section, and most of them should be easily accessible to you.

Breakfast

Before setting out to make your ketogenic breakfast, you should ask yourself: do you want your food to get prepared with minimal cooking or not cooked at all? You can make meals that you can finish up in five minutes, and the good thing is that breakfasts generally cook quickly, so it is a win-win situation. Below are some breakfast ideas that may work for you.

Eggs

The only nutrient that will be missing in your egg meal is a vitamin. It pretty much has all the nutrients that you need, and you can make it by boiling, scrambling, or frying. For a healthy, highly satiating meal, you can choose to add some leafy vegetables as well. You should consider adding other fat sources, such as butter, mayonnaise, or olive oil, to feel full for hours.

If you choose to have breakfast without eggs, there are several other options available for you. You can also try raw nuts, avocados, olives, cheese, smoked salmon, or mackerel. All of these are examples of nutrient-laden meals that you can try, and they are bound to keep you satisfied until lunchtime.

Breakfast Pizza

You do not need pepperoni or cheese to make a keto-friendly pizza. It is a perfect breakfast recipe that uses a cauliflower base and is loaded with avocado, smoked salmon, and runny eggs. With this meal, you can get as much as 7 grams of carbs, together with other nutrients, which makes it a balanced breakfast with coffee or tea.

Collagen Bread

After enjoying this zero-carb bread, you will believe in the existence of miracles. You can either smother it in butter or low-carb strawberry jam or use it as a base for breakfast sandwiches with avocado, fish, bacon or eggs.

Cauliflower Bread with Crispy Bacon, Avocado, and Poached Eggs

Even though most keto cauliflower bread uses

shredded cheese or heavy cream to bind them together, this one is 100% dairy-free. Using a little bit of cauliflower rice and psyllium husk, you can create a hash brown-style base for runny eggs and crispy bacon. It contains about 5.5 grams of net carbs.

Rosemary Bagel

This is another excellent food that is best served after smearing grass-fed butter or stacking meat and eggs on top. The spongy texture of herby bagels comes from a combination of almond flour, xanthan gum, and psyllium husk. The great part is that you can enjoy this keto breakfast recipe at only 9 grams of net carbs per bagel.

Cinnamon Sugar Doughnuts with Almond Flour

These cake-like doughnuts have the perfect crumb and light crunch from a dusting of cinnamon sugar. Having only 3 grams of net carbs per doughnut, you can sneak in an extra one to dunk in your coffee without feeling guilty. You can swap coconut milk for almond milk, as well as utilize grass-fed butter and non-GMO erythritol to make the recipe keto friendly.

Keto Chocolate Doughnuts

Although tender, chocolate-filled doughnuts are perfect on their own, this breakfast recipe gets enhanced with a rich, sweet glaze. You can enjoy them when combined with coffee and tea or eaten as a dessert. With a little over 2 grams of carbs per doughnut, it will not affect your progress if you want to indulge. If you wish to try other varieties, you can make use of grass-fed butter and coffee or change heavy cream with full-fat coconut milk for the glaze.

Classic Bulletproof/Butter Coffee

Bulletproof or butter coffee is an incredible way to begin your day. This recipe is so magical that it causes us to get up in the morning. We have learned not only the official recipe for bulletproof coffee but also the reasons why it works to suppress hunger and how it switches on the brain. It is absolutely carb-free.

Adaptogenic Bulletproof/Butter Coffee

This is a spin on the original bulletproof coffee, which makes use of adaptogens to lift up your mood and help you fight fatigue. Also, the beverage has anti-inflammatory turmeric and vanilla bean that can make the start of your day both sweet and satisfying. This keto breakfast contains about a gram of carbs.

Bulletproof/Butter Coffee Egg Latte

You probably have the urge to exclaim, "Raw eggs? In coffee?" Well, you will never get to find out how tasty this combo is if you do not give it a try. With egg yolk, you get a satisfying creaminess, after all, while healthy fat is added to this keto breakfast recipe. It may also pass as a post-workout drink, considering you consume a gram of carb per mug.

Iced Macha Latte

Despite its cool and creamy nature, an iced matcha latte still delivers a dose of caffeine while supplying healthy fats from coconut milk. Each mug gives about 4.8 grams of net carbs and is an excellent pair for a full plate of bacon.

Anti-Inflammatory Spiced Chai Latte

With earthy turmeric, this recipe contains a golden hue, as well as fuel from fat. It also has gut-healing benefits from gelatin and collagen and is a caffeine-free alternative that's easy on the stomach. It only contains about 3 grams of total carbs.

CBD Rooibos Tea Latte

Cannabidiol (CBD) oil is an optional breakfast recipe, but including it to your diet can be a perfect way to start the day. Caffeine-free rooibos tea gets upgraded with grass-fed ghee, collagen, and CBD oil to create a warm and creamy latte, which is capable of helping you to keep your cool. The best part of it is that it only has a gram of carb per serving.

Fluffy Almond Flour Pancakes

With notes of vanilla and cinnamon, this is a keto breakfast recipe that the entire family can enjoy. Also, it is easy to combine the ingredients. You will first have to blend all the items together and then spoon the batter onto a greased griddle pan. This meal provides about 4.5 grams of net carbs for each serving, and it is the best solution for your pancake cravings.

Coconut Flour Crepes

These light and thin crepes are perfect options to be used as a base for low-sugar berries or coconut whipped cream. To make this breakfast more keto-friendly, you can use water or coconut milk instead of almond milk. This recipe also gives you about a gram of carb per crepe.

Strawberry-Chocolate Crepes

Light and sweet crepes get star treatment from a thick, dark chocolate sauce and chunks of fresh strawberries. Best of all, this indulgent recipe only provides 5 grams of net carbs. Use grass-fed butter (or dairy-free coconut oil) to keep this breakfast bulletproof.

Paleo Chocolate Almond Butter Crepes

Are you running short of berries? There's no need to worry since this keto breakfast has your crepes swimming in a thick almond butter-based chocolate sauce. This meal provides approximately 3 grams of net carbs per filled crepe, and the recipe is straightforward and keto-friendly. Make use of full-fat coconut milk, raw almond butter, or grass-fed butter to make it Bulletproof.

Buttery Coconut Flour Waffles

Mixing coconut flour, non-dairy milk, and eggs can turn into crisp and fluffy waffles. With about 4 grams of net carbs in each waffle, this keto meal makes the perfect addition to a plate of bacon and eggs. To give a bulletproof spin on this recipe, you can make use of full-fat coconut milk and grass-fed butter as your dairy choices

Bacon-and-Egg Fat Bombs

Fat bombs don't need to be too sweet. This savory keto breakfast recipe uses something like an egg salad mixture and surrounds it with bits of crisp bacon for a fun take on the original bacon-and-eggs variety. It contains 2 grams of net carbs and is absolutely keto-friendly. You can make use an avocado oil-based mayo to keep these little bites bulletproof.

Bacon-and-Egg Breakfast Muffins

Egg muffins are the perfect make-ahead keto breakfast to keep you on track. Plus, they're easy to customize. With only 4 grams of net carbs per cup, you can enjoy it either in the morning or during nighttime. You only need to ensure that you use pastured bacon to make it healthier.

Bacon Hash

You can turn chopped cauliflower into a savory potato alternative in this take on a breakfast hash. It only requires 15 minutes to prepare, and it serves as a brilliant option for weekday mornings or weekend brunches. If you wish to make this keto breakfast recipe bulletproof, you only need to use pastured bacon.

Keto Breakfast Wrap

This recipe uses a combination of a layer of egg omelet and avocado in a neat nori sheet so that you can have a breakfast on-the-go. Although the avocado and nori add filling fiber to the meal, the entire meal merely contains 2 grams of net carbs.

Egg Crepes with Avocados

This meal takes a flour-free approach to crepes by using a cooked egg to wrap up layers of mayo, meat, and avocado. You only obtain a gram of carb from one whole crepe. If you are considering to keep it bulletproof, make use of pastured bacon instead of turkey, and then add avocado oil mayo. Cook your egg gently, too.

Lemon Blueberry Muffins

This moist and hearty vanilla cake gets studded with fresh and sweet blueberries. What else can you look for in a keto breakfast recipe? With about 6 grams of carbs per muffin, these glazed bites can become the highlight of your morning.

Dairy-Free Keto Chocolate Muffins

These little cakes stay moist with fiber-filled pumpkin, which turns them into a delicious keto breakfast that is capable of silencing your chocolate cravings. It has added collagen peptides that can smooth your skin and strengthen your hair and nails. You can enjoy all these benefits by merely consuming 3 grams of carbs per muffin.

Crisp Cinnamon Toast Crunch Cereal

You should be excited to see that low-carb cereals have finally arrived. This keto breakfast idea is lovely and munchable, all thanks to a crispy dough that is made from almond flour, warm cinnamon, and grass-fed butter. It contains 2 grams of carbs per serving only and is a significant upgrade from the boxed stuff, taste and nutrition-wise.

Chocolate-Coconut Keto Smoothie Bowl

This is a creamy, dreamy keto breakfast recipe that tastes like dessert and fills your bowl with healthy fat and protein from coconut milk and collagen peptides. It only contains 8 grams of net carbs. Eating this meal will make you feel as good as it looks.

Keto Green Smoothie

Begin your day with a whopping 6 grams of fiber and 8 grams of carbs from a keto green smoothie. This liquid meal combines frozen avocado chunks and a spicy ginger blend together with green veggies for a filling, frosty breakfast substitute. If you desire to stay bulletproof, make use of organic spinach and steam it lightly before adding to your blender.

Low-Carb Cucumber Green Tea Detox Smoothie

This comes with a caffeinated touch from matcha powder and creaminess from the avocado. It is an emerald-colored keto breakfast recipe that is perfect for any morning and not just for detoxification purposes. Make use of high-quality matcha without sweeteners to keep this smoothie bulletproof.

Lunch

Unlike breakfasts, lunchtime meals are not usually as light, and they often require more effort to put together. In this section, we will give you some details about keto-friendly lunch recipes that will make it easier to commit to your health goals than ever.

Loaded Chicken Salad

From golden-brown chicken and lightly grilled asparagus, down to the fresh avocado chunks and creamy spheres of mozzarella, this protein-laden meal is the best keto lunch idea. With every bite, you are bound to get an explosion of flavors in your mouth and always look forward to munching on every last bit of the salad during mealtime.

Zucchini Crust Grilled Cheese

Thanks to the carb-free bread slices that can be made

with mozzarella, parmesan, and grated cheddar sitting right in the middle, grilled cheese isn't here to mess around. There is no need to worry about balance because, in each sandwich, you have two cups of grated zucchini as a part of the bread. Therefore, you can get an ample amount of vegetables along with the cheeses.

Salad with Roasted Cauliflower

It may be quite tasking to be on a keto diet and stay vegan at the same time, but with recipes like the salad with roasted cauliflower, it is not an impossible thing to do. With lots of olive oil, nuts, and avocado to provide those satisfying, healthy fats, the cauliflower becomes better and more pleasing to munch on than leafy greens.

Shrimp Avocado Salad

It takes only 15 minutes to prepare this meal and, within that short period, only five minutes is spent on actual cooking. Once the shrimp is stirred in the butter, you only need to dice the vegetables and make the dressing. It's super easy, fast, and filled with the best flavors.

Keto Chicken Enchilada Bowl

If you are going on a keto diet, make up your mind to become friends with cauliflower. It is the ingredient that makes these meals possible. In place of rice, and topped with some sauced-up chicken, avocado, and cheese, it allows you to stay carb-free while still enjoying an enchilada.

Keto Quesadillas

These are almost exactly like regular tortillas, but the wraps for these cheesy wedges are actually made from mostly eggs and coconut flour. Once the quesadillas win your heart over, feel free to use the tortilla for other dishes like soft tacos.

Sesame Salmon with Baby Bok Choy and Mushrooms

You may need 30 minutes to prepare this meal, but it gets to serve you for as long as the next four lunchtimes, so this is an absolutely time-saving recipe. The longer you let the salmon and vegetables sit in the marinade, the tastier they will become with every day that passes. Be sure that you can use up all the fish by the fourth day to prevent it from going in the trash.

Salmon and Avocado Nori Rolls

Are you used to including sushi on your meals every week before you have decided to go on the keto diet? If your answer is yes, you do not have much to miss out on. You can make keto-friendly rolls, too. All you need to do is to exclude rice from your roll, and then allow the salmon, avocado, and cucumber to play the lead roles.

Caprese Tuna Salad Stuffed Tomatoes

Coated in balsamic vinegar instead of mayo, this Italian-inspired tuna salad is a very viable option for you when you want to take your lunch to work. Stuffed in tomatoes, it's not just a perfect low-carb option. It also scores some points when it comes to the presentation as the colors are appealing to the eyes.

Caprese Eggplant Panini with Lemon Basil Aioli

With your new keto lifestyle, you can increase your vegetable intake in some very creative ways. In this recipe, to be specific, the egg is replaced with eggplant, while the classic Panini goodies like mozzarella, basil, and tomato are tucked inside. You can serve it with creamy garlic aioli. Voila, your gourmet lunch is ready.

Cinnamon Pork Chops and Mock Apples

You may have presumed that pork chops and apples are more suitable for dinner, but that is not entirely true. This meal idea shows how it can be made to become a perfect option even for lunch. Before you object that apples aren't keto-friendly, note that you can use the chayote squash with cinnamon and nutmeg instead of the real fruit.

Spicy Kimchi Ahi Poke

Because your body's still adjusting to the high-fat lifestyle, your digestion may require a bit of nudge. To help it along, you should keep your gut health in check with probiotic-rich foods like kimchi. This fermented cabbage can do wonders for your stomach. When it is mixed with a bit of mayo, tuna, and avocado, it passes for a pretty awesome lunch.

Spinach Mozzarella Stuffed Burgers

Do you want to know how it can be possible for you to contain your cheeseburger fixings without the bread? It's easy. The best advice is to take the Juicy Lucy route. You just need to stuff the greens and the cheese inside the beef patty, instead of piling it on top. Not only does it give you a great taste, but it also makes eating more fun this way.

Low-Carb Mexican Meatza

The traditional pizza might be off-limits for you on the keto diet, but since life without pizza doesn't seem to ever be an option, here's an excellent alternative for you: the low-carb Mexican meatza. The crust is made with cauliflower and has ground beef to give you some protein. Your fat sources in this recipe are the avocado and cheddar toppings, which can supply your ketogenic needs.

Easy Keto Egg Salad

Because the focus of the keto diet is on high-fat and moderate-protein meals, a ketogenic dieter needs a good egg salad recipe up their sleeve. This one is just perfect since it makes use of avocado for extra heart-healthy fatty acids, as well as dill for a boost of fresh flavor.

Low-Carb Chicken Philly Cheesesteak

Do away with the bread and load up on the filling, which is the best part of this chicken Philly cheesesteak-in-a-bowl anyway. With this meal, you have everything you need, from the meat and the Worcestershire sauce to the provolone and the peppers, so you don't ever have to miss the hoagie roll.

Easy Asiago Cauliflower Rice

There are three keywords in this recipe. Cheese. Cream. Rice. Well, this is not precisely rice but riced cauliflower, so once you cook it and coat it with the said cheese and cream, we can guarantee that you'd never be able to tell the difference.

Keto Broccoli Soup with Turmeric and Ginger

Get a thermos and fill it with this creamy, six-ingredient broccoli soup. Thanks to the coconut milk, you will surely leave your taste buds dancing for joy, and the anti-inflammatory turmeric and ginger will make your immune system happy too.

Keto Chili

This make-ahead, slow-cooker chili makes up for the beans that are lacking in your diet. Adding ground sausage with the ground beef makes for a really meaty meal. Just make sure that your tomato paste doesn't have any added sugars because they are absolutely not allowed on the keto diet.

Dinner

After a long day at work, you obviously do not want to come home to a boring meal. Dinners are your last chance to fill up before your day ends. Here are some great ideas to be sure that all your effort throughout the rest of the day is not wasted.

Sesame Chicken

Everyone who is a fan of Chinese food will have some idea of what sesame chicken is, as well as how good it tastes. The problem is that the regular variety will most likely have more carbohydrates in it. To make it keto-friendly, you can have the breaded sesame chicken with a large portion of veggies.

Creamy Chicken Bacon Casserole

If you are a lover of chicken and bacon, imagine how good they will be if you eat them together in a casserole. You can go through this meal for days on end without concern. Note that without some kind of vegetables mixed into it, it will not be a casserole. For this recipe, you will need a pound of broccoli. The latter may prevent the dish from lasting for too long, but there is nothing wrong with devouring leftovers, especially if they taste this good.

Oven-Baked Chicken Avocado Casserole

The good thing about casseroles is that almost no varieties are the same. There are so many combinations of foods that you can combine into one. You can choose to add anything together, throw it in the oven, add some cheese on top, and voila, your casserole is ready. Casseroles are unique because they can have superfoods in them, including avocados, which are one of the healthiest foods on the planet. It's filled with numerous vitamins and minerals that are significant contributors to your overall health. If you like guacamole, then you'll love the taste of a chicken avocado casserole.

Bacon Cheeseburger Casserole

Consider this recipe as something similar to a burger pie. It is going to be slightly time-consuming to make, but it will last you for days, so it is worth your time and effort. If you think you have to eat a lot to keep up with your macros, you'll still have plenty of leftovers to go through, so don't worry about that. In each bite, you will get the taste of a cheeseburger without the bun.

Chicken Cordon Bleu

Consider getting a little fancy by making an oven-baked chicken cordon bleu. If you've never had it in the past, you should know that it comes with a fantastic combination of chicken and ham. Yes, you guessed right: it tastes just as good as it sounds! When the juices from both types of meat mix together, they make for one of the most delicious meals you will ever eat so there will be no surprise when it becomes one of your favorites.

Stuffed Pork Chops

Pork chops are great, but they can get a little boring sometimes if you continue to eat the same type all the time. For this reason, you may consider switching it up a bit. Pork chops are all-time-favorite meals, but what do you think about stuffing them? You have to ensure that you cook the pork all the way through since you cannot prepare a stuffed version in the same way that you make a typical pork chop. That's the way things are, but once you have cooked the pork chops correctly, you will feel fulfilled, knowing that you have prepared a fantastic meal.

Parmesan-Dijon Crusted Pork Chops

When you're able to get an effective breading on your protein aside from breadcrumbs, you will have to take advantage of this recipe. Adding breading to anything is going to give a bit of crunch that may be missing in other recipes. You will, therefore, be happily surprised with how your recipe turns out.

Keto Lime Pork Chops

Although you might initially think that the lime flavor doesn't go well with pork chops, you should not knock the idea out until you try it. You'll discover that the combination works surprisingly well.

Creamy Mustard Lemon Pork

If you want a slice of tender pork that is filled with flavor, cooking creamy mustard lemon pork is always a great idea. Perfecting this recipe will give you a tender piece of meat that will gently melt in your mouth with every bite you take. Try not to drool over yourself when the recipe turns out well.

Cumin-Spiced Beef Wraps

These beef wraps can act as either a full meal or a quick snack, depending on the amount you choose to make. Though the recipe comes in 8 wraps, it counts for just 2 servings. The wraps themselves will be lettuce, which is perfect for this keto diet. It may not have the same consistency as a regular tortilla or something similar, but the taste is going to come out almost the same. Lettuce wraps replace flour tortillas, and there will be no regretting it.

Cheeseburger Calzone

If you love calzones and/or cheeseburgers, then you will need to try this recipe. A big, meaty calzone that tastes like a cheeseburger is something that some people may consider a dream, but this recipe proves that it can happen. One of the best parts about this cheeseburger calzone is that, when made correctly, you can get up to 8 servings. This meal can last you for one week or a few days, depending on how often you munch on it.

Swedish Meatballs

Who doesn't love to have a good meatball from time to time? Even if you don't like meatballs, give this recipe a try because it tastes that good and you deserve to have it. Meatballs will go with almost anything, and this Swedish recipe is perfect for you.

Stuffed and Wrapped Shrimp

Shrimp is one of our favorite keto-friendly meals. When great flavors are added to an already delicious entree, your taste buds may pop up gleefully to thank you. This recipe for jalapeno stuffed shrimp wrapped in bacon is easy to follow. Since the bacon doesn't take too long to cook, you can have a delicious meal waiting for you in a few minutes.

Shrimp Scampi

When starting with the keto diet, you need to tap into the recipes that remind you of the menu that you used to be on before starting the new one. We are specifically talking about dishes that will remind you of carbohydrates, such as shrimp scampi. Using zucchini, though, you will make a meal of noodles, which looks similar to regular noodles. This way, it may feel like you are eating the real version of the dish.

Salmon Curry

Did you know that you can make an excellent curry dish with seafood? The salmon curry is absolutely a must-try for those who enjoy curry. You can easily replace the rice with riced cauliflower or other riced veggies.

Seafood Soup

Generally, seafood is great for the keto diet. Nevertheless, it is going to taste even better when put in soup, regardless of the broth used. Since it incorporates both seafood and broth, you probably won't mind sipping it all day.

Chapter 6: Intermittent Fasting

Intermittent fasting has become a new craze in the world of fitness. According to theories, it helps people to stay fit, live longer, and even lose weight. Unlike the ketogenic diet, intermittent fasting is not a diet plan since it does not provide restrictions to what you eat. It practically focuses on a modern approach to eating and fasting. There are many health benefits to this dietary plan, including weight loss. However, before starting it, you should find out if it is suitable for you since it is not always a healthy choice for everybody. In summary, intermittent fasting, unlike other weight-loss therapies, is a pattern that circles around the way you eat, regardless of your food choices.

Although there is no standard duration for fasting, the most common intermittent fasts involve fasting for 16 hours every day or 24 hours two times a week. Whenever you find yourself not eating, you are fasting. This can take place between breakfast and lunch or lunch and dinner. Naturally, humans are wired to be able to function for long hours without food. In fact, history proves that ancient hunters could carry on for days in the wild without food, as they couldn't preserve it for consumption later. This made them have to fast until they could get something to eat again. Fasting for religious purposes is also seen in modern society. Fasting is seen as a more natural phenomenon than that of the practice of eating three to four times daily and can be taken as a part of everyday life.

There is a need to distinguish fasting from starvation since some people may think that they are the same thing. Fasting is a controlled absence of food for a specific goal and gain, which may be spiritual or health-related. Starvation is the involuntary absence of food, which eventually leads to suffering and even death. The former is usually done by people who have enough body fats stored to carry them through for a specific period. It is not recommended for underweight people and does not in any way lead to suffering and or death. When fasting, food is available, but the dieter chooses to do without it for some hours, days, and even weeks, depending on how long they can go without eating. You may choose to start or stop fasting at any time.

Even though intermittent fasting is currently gaining widespread recognition across the globe, it is not as new as people may realize. Fasting has been in existence for centuries now. It is probably the most potent and oldest dietary intervention in the history of man; however, it has been overlooked and relegated. To get the best results out of this method, you should familiarize yourself with everything there is to know about it.

How Intermittent Fasting Works for Weight Loss

When you engage in intermittent fasting, your body begins to use its stored fat as a source of energy. It is the reason that you can typically function for hours without food. This means that, when you fast, your body burns excess fat and keeps you from feeling hungry. The fact is that fasting and eating are opposite of each other. At any point, you can choose to either eat or fast. When you eat, your body gets more energy than it actually needs, while the insulin level rises immediately. With the help of insulin, the excess fat in the body gets stored away to be used at a later time. It also allows the storage of carbohydrates into individual glucose units, which are linked with long-chain glycogen, which is later stored in the liver. For biological reasons, there is hardly enough space in the liver to store glycogen. Once the limit is reached, therefore, the body automatically transforms excess glucose into fat. This process is known as de novo lipogenesis, which means "making new fat." While some of the newly created fat is stored in the liver, others get deposited in other parts of the body. Although this is a complicated process, there is absolutely no limit to the amount of fat that can be produced naturally.

During intermittent fasting, there is a drastic fall in the level of insulin in your body, thus sending a signal to your entire system to notify your body parts of the scarcity of energy from food. This makes you experience a drop in the level of blood glucose, forcing the body to go to the storage facilities to get energized. Glycogen, which is the most accessible source of energy, is in limited supply. It can only last for about 24 to 36 hours. Once the stored glycogen is exhausted, your body is then forced to break down the stored fat to get energy. This means that your body survives in either the fed state, which is the insulin-high state, or the fasted state, which is the insulin-low state. The former contributes to weight gain because if, say, if you spend your entire day eating, there will be no room for the body to burn fat from the stored reserves. It is necessary for your body to strike a balance between the fed state and the fasted state so that it can burn stored fat and allow you to lose weight. This is precisely what intermittent fasting does, and there is absolutely nothing wrong with it. As mentioned above, it is how our bodies are wired. If you continue to eat without resting, the body will always have glycogen to use. This causes it to keep storing what you eat as fat until you have nothing to eat. That's the only time when it can burn the excess fat. Without ever being in the fasted state, there will never be a need for your body to consume stored fat so you will keep gaining weight.

Although some benefits come with intermittent fasting, aside from religious purposes, weight loss is the main reason why people fast. While fasting, you eat fewer meals, leading to an automatic reduction in the level of calories. It also changes the levels of hormones that aid in weight loss. It causes an increase in the level of fat-burning hormones norepinephrine or noradrenaline. These changes in hormones contribute to the rise in the metabolic rate of the body by 3.6-14%. The caloric equation is also affected on both sides to create a balance by helping you during intermittent fasting by eating fewer calories while burning more of them. According to a study, this fast makes people lose muscle than other known standard methods (Gunnars, 2016). Eating large amounts of food during this period may increase your caloric level and have the opposite effect that you are aiming for.

Several benefits attached to intermittent fasting include, overall health improvement, increased brain condition, can reduce the risk of developing type 2 diabetes, cancer, and heart-related diseases.

Science Behind Intermittent Fasting

To dissect the science behind intermittent fasting, we will take a quick look at the history of the dietary pattern, which experts say dates back to as far as two million years ago. It is theorized to begin during the evolution of the genus homo, that we humans are evolved from, whom anthropologists believe to be hunters. This is how it worked at the time: when a band of hunters killed game that they found, it meant that they had a bounty of a calorie-rich diet. At the end of the feast, they were left to survive on herbs, cereal grains, and roots that had little to no calories at all. After agriculture was invented by humans about ten thousand years ago, there is now a predictable and surplus supply of calories. Fast forward to modern times, and us humans have been able to maximize survival capacity through a metabolic and biochemical food selection process in times of food-related crises, such as famines and scarcity of food. This is why humans now have tendencies of being plump and even obese. The reason behind the overweight trends, however, lies in the psychology of modern times. Our metabolic standpoint has become higher than when our ancestors had to survive on hunting and gathering to survive. Scientifically speaking, there have not been a significant amount of changes in the metabolic processes of Homo sapiens sapiens, which are geared towards conserving energy related to uneven caloric reserves. Due to food intake restrictions by our ancestors, the body developed a means to maintain its functions. This is essential for the body to adapt perfectly in times when you change your diet. Our modern world has made food varieties available, and we get to eat what we want anytime. In fact, many health practitioners have advised that people should spread their meals to 5 or 6 different times a day. The body sees this as a food surplus, which affects its ability to repair vital tissues that should slow down the aging process.

Consequently, the hormones charged with the responsibility of maintaining the physiological stability now resists changes in the set metabolic point. This is a phenomenon that is known to everyone who has ever gone on a diet. Also, theorists say that there is a problem with our gut flora, a community of microorganisms that live in the digestive tracts of humans and animals. According to experts, obesity causes a change in the gut where the new flora now promotes weight gain. This was probably not the case for people millennia ago.

Researchers from the Salk Institute went into an investigation and found that the method is not totally devoid of problems. According to a study done on mice, when food was withdrawn from them for 24 hours, 90% of the internal organs that are under the control of the circadian regulation ceased to function (Micheali, 2017). This isn't a remarkable feat as it is expected that the main metabolic organs will be primarily influenced by the amount of food. The study, however, also revealed that when the mice were placed on a high-fat diet, most of the organs became extremely active. As a result, the mice were reported to have become obese. This practically explains the science/mechanism behind intermittent fasting and feeding on a molecular level. There is still no conclusive research regarding the full extent of the benefits of intermittent fasting in humans.

Dr. Krysta Varady of the Illinois University in Chicago (2015) carried out a research on 86 obese women and 14 obese men (a total of 100 people), spread through three random groups, for a whole year. They were asked to observe alternate-day fasts, supplying them with 25% of their energy needs on fast days and 125% energy needs on eating days. As for calorie supplies, 75% of the caloric needs were supplied daily in some days, and there were no caloric restrictions at all on other days. This trial, however, involved phases of weight loss and gain for six months each. The result revealed that the alternate-day fasting did not produce superior adherence to weight loss, cardioprotection, or maintenance, as opposed to caloric restriction. Varady stated in an interview that the efficacy of intermittent fasting does not lay in any adaptation theory of evolution as propagated by historians or a complicated genetic, molecular mechanism. It rather lies in tricking/training your mind and body to eat less. As a result of weight loss, the body gets all the metabolic benefits. This simply means that the method works not because of what goes on within us scientifically but because of the food that we eat, which is mainly characterized by how we consume it.

Effects of Intermittent Fasting on Cells and Hormones

During fasting, the body is exposed to several cellular and molecular activities. It needs to adjust and make stored fats more accessible. Below are some of the things that happen in the body during intermittent fasting.

1. Increases human growth hormones

The level of growth hormones, which is multiplied as much as five times, shoots up. It improves the loss of fat and increases the gains of muscle mass.

2. Improves insulin sensitivity

When you fast, the levels of insulin in your body drops drastically while improving insulin sensitivity. The lower the insulin level is, the easier it is to access the fat that has been stored in your system.

3. Repairs cells

When you are fasting, the body automatically initiates a process called autophagy that repairs cells. The digestion of old and dysfunctional proteins that have been stored inside the cell also takes place.

4. Expresses genes

The genes that are related to longevity also undergo some changes and experience protection against diseases.

5. Reduces inflammation

Some studies have noted a drastic reduction in some inflammation markers, which are vital contributors to various chronic diseases.

6. Prevents cancer

According to a study on animals, intermittent fasting can be a great contributor to the reduction or prevention of cancer (Gunnars, 2016).

7. Improves brain health

The brain hormone BDNF is increased by intermittent fasting, leading to the growth of new nerve cells. It also contributes to protecting against Alzheimer's disease.

8. Promotes anti-aging

Studies say that intermittent fasting can increase the lifespan of rats that have been used in some research. It showed that the rats that were placed on the fast had chances of living 80% longer.

Methods of Intermittent Fasting

Thankfully, the intermittent fast is a natural regimen that can be done in whichever way you want. For more extended fasting periods, it is advised that the fast should be done under the supervision of a health practitioner. On a general note, shorter fasts are the most commonly practiced. There are several ways that you can try fasting intermittently, but you are expected to split days or weeks into periods of both eating and fasting on all of them. During the fasting periods, though, you may either eat very little or eat nothing at all.

The most popular fasting methods are:

16/8 Method

This technique also called the Lean Gains protocol. You are required to fast for 16 hours. It is sometimes also known as the 8-hour eating window. Here, all your meals are eaten within 8 hours, while you avoid food of any kind in the remaining 16 hours. With this method, you simply skip breakfast, eat the other meals within the 8-hour window, and fast for the rest of the day. Although most people do not eat in the morning, others prefer to skip dinner. Typically, the technique involves eating two to three meals daily. On this fast, you can drink as many zero-calorie beverages as you want.

Eat-Stop-Eat

This fasting method entails that you should not eat anything for 24 hours twice a week. It is a technique that has been introduced by Brad Pilon. Without any form of restrictions, the only rule is that you must fast for 24 hours and that the fasting must not be done on two consecutive days. It is not advisable for people who are not used to skipping meals. It can be absolutely impossible for some people to stay away from foods for 24 hours. They tend to feel extremely hungry during that period, to the extent that these folks might become irritable and unable to function normally.

Warrior Diet

This is a fasting method introduced by Ori Hofmekler, and it entails that people should eat a small amount of food within 20 hours daily. This method requires you to eat all of your meals in the remaining 24 hours of the day. This, however, may not be a simple technique to try as the consumption of a large amount of food may not settle well with your stomach. It is regarded as the most extreme fasting method and cannot be recommended to people who are barely getting used to fasting.

Alternate-Day Fasting (5/2 Method)

The technique is used to improve blood sugar, calorie, and cholesterol levels by fasting on alternate days. With the 5/2 method, you're expected to eat 500 to 600 calories on two non-consecutive days every week. For some people, an extra day is added every week. For the remaining days of the week, the individual should merely consume the same number of calories that he or she has burned during the day. The result is that there will be a deficiency in calories over time so that you begin to lose weight.

Exercising During Intermittent Fasting

If you are fasting and still want to continue your workout routines, there are some things you must consider before doing so. Those who are fasting to lose weight, the good news is that when fasting and exercise are combined, you have a higher possibility of dissolving more fats. While some research says that combining fasting and exercise affects the biochemistry and metabolism of the muscles that are linked with insulin sensitivity and the control of blood sugar levels, others support exercising immediately after eating before the occurrence of digestion and absorption. This is said to be essential for people suffering from type 2 diabetes and metabolic syndrome. The good thing about fasting is that glycogen is likely depleted during fasting so you will burn more fat to fuel your exercise. Other studies have countered this research, though, claiming that people do not burn more by exercising on an empty stomach. If you think that exercising while fasting is a good idea, you may want to consider some of its downsides (Weatherspoon, 2018).

Working out and fasting at the same time can lead to the loss of muscles. Because of that, you may be able to maintain your muscles, but you cannot gain more. Your body can break down tissues and use their protein as energy during intermittent fasting. This means is that you will have limited power to work out as hard or perform as well as you usually do on a regular diet. There is also a chance of you falling or hitting a wall. Another theory states that the body reduces its calories and energy, so it may end up slowing down your metabolic processes.

Tips for Combining Intermittent Fasting with Exercise

If you are convinced that your body genuinely needs a combination of intermittent fasting and exercise, here are some things you may want to try to get the best out of both regimens.

1. Think about timing critically

Christopher Shuff (2018), a dietician, says that there are three things to consider in order to make workout effective while fasting. He states that you should consider whether he or she wants to exercise during, before or after the fueling window. One of the most common methods of combining exercise with intermittent fasting is the Lean Gains 16:8 protocol. For someone who can function well when exercising on an empty stomach, working out before the timeframe is an ideal option. If you do not like to work out on an empty stomach, doing it during the window is best. This is also a good option because you get to tap into all the post-workout nutrition. Shuff, however, explains that exercising while fasting is beneficial when it comes to recovery and performance. Working out after the window, therefore, is for those who prefer to work out with a satiated stomach but do not have the chance to do so during the eating period.

2. Select workout types based on your macros

According to experts, it is crucial to pay attention to the macronutrients that you eat during the day before and after your workout session. For example, having a high amount of carbohydrates is essential for strength training, while eating a small number of carbs can be acceptable when you are doing high-intensity interval training (HIIT).

3. Build or maintain muscles

You should build or keep muscles by eating the right foods after exercising. The best option for the individuals who wish to combine working out with intermittent fasting is to time the fitness periods so that they correlate with eating periods to ensure that nutrition levels are at their peak. For someone who lifts heavy weights, it is a good idea to eat protein after a workout session to aid in muscle regeneration. It is advised to consume approximately 20 grams of protein within 30 minutes post-workout.

As you may already know, the success of any exercise or weight-loss regimen depends on its safety and sustainability over time. If you intend to lose weight while maintaining your fitness level during intermittent fasting, you should try to stay in the safe zone as much as possible.

- **Eat a meal close to your workout**: Having your meal at a time when your moderate or high-intensity exercise is close is very important. By doing so, there will be glycogen available for your body to tap into to gain energy.

- **Stay hydrated**: Always keep in mind that even if you are fasting, it does not mean that you should avoid drinking water. As a matter of fact, it is during this time that you need more water than ever. Therefore, you are advised to drink lots of water when fasting, and even more so when you fast and exercise simultaneously.
- **Keep your electrolytes up**: Be mindful of sports drinks during workouts because most of them are high in sugar. You should try to avoid them as much as you can. A good substitute for such beverages is coconut water, which is a high-caloric source of hydration. While it replenishes the electrolytes in your body, it also provides a low amount of calories.
- **Combine low-intensity workouts with short workout time**: If you are engaging in the 24-hour intermittent fast, try to carry out low-intensity workouts, such as restorative yoga and walking. When doing the other types, you may stick with regular exercise routines.

- **Listen to your body**: Finally, the best thing to do when working out during an intermittent fast is to listen to your body. You will know when you have reached your limit and can no longer push forward further. If, for example, you begin to feel weak or dizzy, it is a clear sign that you have either become dehydrated or experienced a drop in your blood sugar level. In cases like this, you are advised to drink electrolytes immediately and then eat a well-balanced meal as soon as possible.

In a nutshell, while the combination of intermittent fasting and exercise may be an excellent idea for some people, it's not ideal for others who need to stay away from any strenuous activity while fasting. Whatever the situation may be, it is always good to check with a healthcare expert before engaging in any exercise or nutritional activity.

Enjoying this book so far? I'd love it for you to share your thoughts and post a quick review on Audible!

Chapter 7: Benefits of Intermittent Fasting

Weight Loss

Considering many people who go on the fast do so for the sole purpose of losing weight, this is the most popular benefit of intermittent fasting. The popularity of the method has been gaining more ground in recent years as a result of its efficacy in promoting weight loss. Fasting pushes the body to shed a few pounds by bringing down insulin levels (a hormone that allows cells to take in glucose). Typically, the system breaks carbohydrates down to glucose, which is later used by cells for energy, or converted into fat and stored in the body for future use. During the times when you are not eating, there is usually a drop in the levels of insulin. The depleting insulin levels cause cells to release the stored glucose as energy. The repetition of this process, which takes place during intermittent fasting, may lead to the loss of weight. Not to mention, the consumption of a fewer amount of calories can cause a reduction in weight. Though it may not be more effective than other traditional techniques that are based on caloric restrictions, intermittent fasting is doable for people who want to start shedding some pounds.

Reduction in the Risk Type 2 Diabetes

Together with its weight loss benefits, intermittent fasting is also useful when it comes to reducing the risk of having or worsening type 2 diabetes. To be specific, it influences other factors that are linked to the condition.

According to health experts, obesity is one of the things that contribute to the development of type 2 diabetes. A 2014 study that has been published in the journal called Translation Research has stated that intermittent fasting can lower blood glucose and insulin levels in people who are at the risk of developing diabetes. Other researches back it up by claiming that fasting is a promising therapy for weight loss and diabetes (Kandola, 2018).

When further studies were conducted to adults who suffer from obesity, it was discovered that there were reductions in diabetes markers (such as sensitivity to insulin), so experts believe that the fast can be useful in the reduction of the disease among this group. On the contrary, a 2018 research conducted on rats showed that intermittent fasting could be capable of increasing the risk of diabetes (Ana, 2018). By tracking the well-being of rodents for three months, it later came out that despite the reduction in weight and food eaten, the abdominal fat tissue increased while the muscle structure decreased - a clear sign of the body not making proper use of insulin. All of these are risk factors of type 2 diabetes (Kandola, 2018). This study, therefore, gives rise to the need for it to be replicated in humans to find out if the results apply to us as well.

Brain Health

As people get older, there is a limited flow of blood to the brain. Neurons shrink, and there is a decline in the amount of brain volume. Luckily, intermittent fasting is capable of stalling the aging process by improving the alertness and overall mental health of humans. Some benefits of intermittent fasting to the brain are:

1. Lowering the risk of brain diseases

Intermittent fasting is capable of boosting the health of your mind by reducing the risk of neurodegenerative diseases such as Alzheimer's and Parkinson's. It is imperative when it comes to the prevention of diabetes and obesity, considering both conditions contribute to the development of Alzheimer's disease.

2. Promotes autophagy and prevents neural degeneration

Another benefit of intermittent fasting is that it assists the brain in preventing the degeneration of nerve cells. According to a 2003 study, the neurons in the brain can be protected against excitotoxic stress, which later leads to neural death, thanks to intermittent fasting (Moodie). Autophagy, which is the process that the brain goes through to get rid of damaged cells and produce new ones, is also boosted by the method. This allows the body to defend itself against various illnesses naturally.

3. Improves memory

It has also been found that intermittent fasting is capable of boosting learning and memory retention.

This is another potent protection against neurodegenerative diseases. Using their ability to recall words, a study carried out in 50 aged people found a boost of memory after getting placed on caloric restriction for three months (Moodie, n.d.).

4. Alleviates depression

Intermittent fasting may also be beneficial for people who deal with mood disorders like depression. According to research in 2013, depressed individuals reported improvements in mental alertness and mood and experienced a sense of peace when they fasted (Moodie).

Longevity

Studies have proven that intermittent fasting helps to guard the body against terminal diseases. Someone devoid of cancer, cardiovascular disease, or diabetes, therefore, is bound to live longer.

1. Lowering cholesterol levels

A study that was carried out in 2010 showed that the overweight women who fasted intermittently showed improvements in some risk factors for chronic diseases (Moodie, n.d.). This includes lowered cholesterol, reduced blood pressure, as well as decreased level of insulin resistance.

2. Slowing down cancer

When combined with chemotherapy, intermittent fasting is also capable of slowing down the progress of skin and other forms of cancer by increasing the level of tumor-infiltrating lymphocytes. These are the cells sent by the immune system to fight the tumor.

3. Making cells resistant

The manipulation of mitochondrial networks is also a way for intermittent fasting to improve your lifespan and slow down the aging process. Mitochondria is the powerhouse - the power generator - of a cell. For the cells to survive, they rely on this organ to provide all the energy they need. A study conducted by Harvard researchers in 2017, however, showed that fasting helped to keep the mitochondria networks together by keeping them healthy enough to process energy effectively. The latter is vital to aging and longevity.

Inflammation Reduction

We are confronted with inflammation in one way or another every day. This can take place if you kick a stone accidentally or get cut from a knife while preparing your family's dinner. It can be the result of a fungus that triggers allergies. When inflammation graduates to a chronic condition, it can lead to excess belly fats and weight gain.

Intermittent fasting has proven to be a handy tool to combat this situation. By not eating, the body produces an anti-inflammatory effect on the body's neurological and immune systems. This is a process that can't happen when you consume meals that are high in carbohydrates. When combined with the keto diet, intermittent fasting can help rid the body of inflammation and its effects.

Immune Regulation

Intermittent fasting forces the body's immune system to perform in peak condition. The majority of the body's energy will help fight off disease. Two major cytokines foster vital inflammatory responses: interleukin-6 and tumor necrosis factor alpha. When you fast, you restrict the release of such molecules.

When you fast intermittently and drink more water and other cleansing beverages, the effect is usually superb. The reason is that this activity cleanses your digestive system, which reduces your gut microbes that affect your immune system.

Insulin Sensitivity Enhancement

Intermittent fasting is a useful tool to improve cellular insulin sensitivity. This allows the body to make effective use of insulin so that it requires less of this chemical after eating. With reduced demand for insulin, the inflammation level reduces and bumps up the body's HGH levels. Insulin and human growth hormone (HGH) work in diverse ways in the body. The former triggers the storage of energy while boosting cellular division and inflammation. The primary assignment of the latter is to encourage tissue repair while at the same time. Between the two, insulin is more valuable. When we consume foods that are rich in starch and carbs, insulin is required to suppress the level of HGH.

During periods of food scarcity, the sensitivity of the body's cell membrane to insulin increases. This is expected - and quite significant - because it makes the body utilize every chunk of food that goes in it. When there is more than enough food, on the other hand, the opposite happens. The body, in a bid to dodge the stress of excessive calorie intake, reduces its sensitivity to insulin. It leads to an increase in insulin level, which then results in excess body fats, inflammatory conditions, and oxidative stress.

Intermittent Fasting and Chronic Diseases

Intermittent fasting has been known to bring about splendid improvements in patients and victims of chronic autoimmune diseases, such as Crohn's, ulcerative colitis, rheumatoid arthritis, and systemic lupus. This is because intermittent fasting tends to reduce the effect of inflammation that causes these illnesses and leads to a normal function of the body's immune system.

Cancer cells, for instance, contains between ten and seventy other insulin receptors more than the average cell. This is the result of the breakdown of sugar, which serves as the body's energy source. When you are fasting intermittently, the body does not get the fuel (sugar) it requires for this disintegration. Thus, cells with free radicals can be destroyed.

While there is a lot of research being conducted regarding the effects of intermittent fasting, experts say that the results are yet to be conclusive. It may take a while before doctors can recommend this technique for clinical use. There is not enough evidence to support some of the claims made by propagators of the theory. It is an established fact that fasting can contribute to weight loss. Also, although many experiments have been carried out on animals, based on the hypothesis of the intermittent fast, most of these researches are yet to be transitioned from animals to humans.

Chapter 7: Intermittent Fasting in Men vs. Women

While it is all right for everyone to observe intermittent fasting, some studies have shown that the results of the fast may not be the same in some women as it is in men. According to research, controlling the blood sugar became more difficult for the females than the males three weeks after they began fasting intermittently (Coyle, 2018). There are also many claims made by women, who believe that their menstrual cycle had changed when they started intermittent fasting. These shifts are tied to the sensitivity of the female population to calorie restrictions.

When there is a low level of calorie due to long hours of fasting or frequent fasting, a part of the brain, which is known as the hypothalamus, is affected. This disrupts the hormone that releases gonadotropin. This hormone further releases two reproductive hormones, which are known as the luteinizing hormone (LH) and the follicle-stimulating hormone (FSH). When there is a breach of communication between these hormones and the ovaries, women run the risk of experiencing irregular menstruations, poor bone health, infertility, and other health complications. Though studies in animals have not been replicated in humans, a research carried out on rats showed that they experienced a reduction in the size of their ovaries when they were placed on three to six months of alternate-day fasting. Irregular reproductive cycles were also some of the side effects of the fast in female rats (Coyle, 2018). These are several reasons why it is advised for women to consider a modified approach to intermittent fastings, such as shorter fasting periods and fewer fasting days. In short, fasting methods that women follow should be less intense than their male counterparts. It is important to note that metabolism and the human reproductive system are deeply interwoven. When a woman misses her period, it is evident that there has been some form of disturbance in her hormones. The hormones that affect a woman's reproductive health are not only restricted to the sex hormones. The ones that store fat as well as in burning it contributes to that process. Because of this, any hormonal imbalance that a woman may experience will likely reflect in her reproductive system.

The less frequent eating pattern that is characterized by intermittent fasting means that you eat less protein. The lack of protein causes negative impacts on women's fertility rate. Stress is your system's antagonist as it raises your cortisol levels and inhibits the production of gonadotropin-releasing hormone, which hinders the ovaries from generating estrogen and progesterone. In truth, the latter is usually converted to cortisol during periods of stress to help the body to cope. This may either prevent weight loss or contribute to weight gain. The singular fact that you eat little food during the fasting stresses out the body as well.

In general, anything capable of affecting reproductive health will also affect weight management, fitness, and well-being, as well as your overall health. If you think intermittent fasting is becoming stressful, you may want to consider that it probably isn't suitable for you. These are some of the reasons why women are advised to try the less stressful versions of the method and take notes of the way their body responds to it.

During the fasting period, pay close attention to the following signs and discontinue the fast if you develop any of them: menstrual irregularities, insomnia, hair loss, slow recovery after injury, acne/rashes, low libido, mood swings, palpitations, sluggish digestion, reduced tolerance to stress, or feeling cold constantly. Intermittent fasting is not recommended to anyone pregnant, suffering or recovering from an eating disorder, battling insomnia, on medication for a chronic condition, under severe stress, depressed, or dealing with any form of severe illness, unless under the direct supervision of a medical professional.

Intermittent Fasting Modifications for Women

If you wish to attempt to try intermittent fasting as a woman, there are some alterations you should make to the plan to make it less strict compared to the standard versions that work for men. While doing this, she will need to consider hunger signals. She can be sure that they are not caused by simple eating habits or boredom; whenever her body indicates the need for food, it is not just merely showing the sign for the fun of it. Chances are, it needs something important, and the consequences of turning a blind eye to it may not be pleasant. Here are some of the things that women can do to make intermittent fasting suitable for them.

Eat Healthy Fats

As you already know, fat isn't something that should be avoided. Essential fatty acids must be part of your diet, in fact, to fight inflammation and improve mental health, among others. When you choose to eat healthy fats, i.e., grass-fed butter, and coconut oil, not only will there be significant work in progress within the body, but there will also be a feeling of satisfaction. You may choose to rely solely on fats during this time without fear of interrupting the body's state of ketosis since you will surely receive enough calories even during this brief eating period.

Choose Low-Impact Foods

Intermittent fasting allows the digestive tract to recuperate and rebuild. This can be supported and given a boost when you choose to consume low-impact foods instead of subjecting yourself to a complete fast. Some common foods that suit this purpose are steamed vegetables, nutritionally rich green powder, and fruits.

Reduce Your Fasting Period

While sleeping, the body naturally goes into a fasting period. This gets broken in the morning once you wake up. This nightly fast can be extended for longer hours, possibly until noon, instead of farther into the day. This way, you will be giving your body a chance to ease the fast into your daily routine without putting in more effort or going through more stress.

Whether you are one of those women whom intermittent fasting works for, or you belong to the group needs to alter their habits drastically, you should find other ways to apply the fasting principles. By paying attention to your body's signals, you will be able to prepare for potential health risks ahead of time. This enables you to look for the best options for your body while staying away from things that may be detrimental to your overall well-being. Like every other dietary program, you should always keep a close watch at methods that work for you as an individual. We have already covered that there is no one-size-fits-all approach to dieting. The fact that a particular method is beneficial for other women does not necessarily mean that it will work in the same way for you.

Chapter 8: Intermittent Fasting and Ketogenic Diet

Intermittent fasting and the ketogenic diet are two of the most recent trends among the health-conscious crowd. Many benefits come from both programs, and many types of research have been done to back them up. While they are best known for controlling weight, that's not all that these two techniques can do. With the growing popularity surrounding these trends, many people are curious as to if these weight-loss methods can be implemented together without possible side effects. The idea of combining both practices is welcome but not absolutely necessary.

If you are one of those individuals who is considering combining both practices, there is good news for you: you can easily follow both of them simultaneously without having to face severe consequences.

Some of the reasons why following the keto diet and intermittent fasting can be right for you are:

1. It makes it easier for your body to reach ketosis.

Adding fasting to your regimen may jumpstart the process of ketosis. This is because the body maintains a balance of energy by shifting its source of fuel from carbs to fat, which is the specific premise of the keto diet. When you fast, your insulin and glycogen levels drop and trigger the burning of fats automatically to maintain enough energy. The combination of both techniques is, therefore, suitable for those people who cannot reach ketosis when only following the ketogenic diet. It may be quicker for your body to enter ketosis when you combine a keto diet with intermittent fasting than merely doing either individually.

2. You may not experience cravings.

When on a keto diet, there is no fear of fat spiking your blood sugar levels. After all, we know by now that fat stabilizes blood sugar. This is so effective that it has been recorded to cure individuals with type 2 diabetes and get them totally off of medication. Combining keto diet and fasting can reduce your blood sugar level without causing you to feel uncomfortable. You can now say goodbye to programs that make you feel awkward with high-carb fasting and induced cravings, fatigue, and mood swings.

3. It helps suppress your hunger.

The ketogenic diet is also very useful in keeping hunger at bay. The liver turns fat stores into ketone energy bundles while you are on the plan. These organic compounds are sent as fuel through the bloodstream. As a result, the ghrelin levels get suppressed during the ketogenic diet. Ghrelin, the primary hunger hormone of the body is suppressed to a minimal level, even when there is no food in your system. Thanks to them, you may not be as hungry as you usually are when you are on a regular weight-loss journey. This causes you to go for hours without feeling famished. That is a definite advantage while you are intermittent fasting. You can then stay on the fast for more extended periods to assist your body in shedding even more pounds.

4. It leads to more fat loss.

You are more likely to burn fat when you combine the fast and the diet than when you are on the diet alone. Simply because intermittent fasting boosts metabolism by promoting thermogenesis or heat production. During thermogenesis, the body automatically begins to search out those stubborn fat stores that are ordinarily inaccessible to start turning those deposits into energy. It is no longer new that intermittent fasting is capable of reducing excess body fat. According to a study that was carried out in 34 resistance-trained men for eight weeks, the ones who practiced the 16:8 fasting method lost approximately 14% more body fat than those who followed the regular dietary pattern. In the same light, the men who supported the low-carb diet lost about 3.3 kilograms (7.3 lbs) of fat mass than the people who followed the proper low-calorie diet (Kubala, 2018). Intermittent fasting also preserves muscle mass when you are losing weight, as well as improving your energy level. This is helpful to those keto dieters who are looking for ways to enhance their athletic performance while continuing to drop some unwanted extra weight.

5. It helps you avoid the side effects of ketosis.

The ketogenic diet can make your fasting periods more natural and more manageable than ever before. For example, when you consume a high amount of carbohydrates while fasting, the fast will cause you to be uncomfortable as your body struggles to make the switch between glucose and ketones for fuel. Eating keto meals during fasting, however, will allow your system to run on ketones whenever you want it to.

If you are either not used to the keto diet or merely starting back up after a break, it is advisable for you to start your journey again with intermittent fasting. This will help you to avoid some of the adverse side effects that you might experience during the early stages of the program, particularly the keto flu. Which you already know is brought on as a result in the drop of glucose levels in the blood while it is switching its use from regular carbohydrates and proteins as their source of energy to ketones from fat.

6. It helps autophagy to work better.

Intermittent fasting activates something called autophagy in the body. This is a state where the body eats its own cells and tissues in an attempt to keep the body healthy. Through this process, the body cleanses itself by getting rid of harmful and toxic substances and recycles damaged proteins. Autophagy operations happen under two conditions: 1) when the body is starved, and 2) when there are restrictions in protein and carbohydrate levels. Because both of these processes take place in both ketogenic dieting and intermittent fasting, their combination will help you reap all the benefits of autophagy healthily and efficiently.

For the majority of people, combining intermittent fasting and the keto diet is a perfectly safe and healthy thing to do. However, as mentioned in other chapters, we want to emphasize that it might not be suitable for everyone. Pregnant women and those who have suffered from an eating disorder are advised to stay away from intermittent fasting. As well as those individuals who are dealing with diabetes or heart-related diseases should consult their doctor before subjecting themselves to either method of losing weight.

Although it might be helpful for some people to combine both practices, you should first find out if it is compatible with your system to know if it's even worth pursuing or not. Besides the possibility of following both techniques being too risky health-wise for some, others may begin to experience adverse side effects, such as overeating during non-fasting days, irritability, and even fatigue. You should always remember that although intermittent fasting is capable of making you reach ketosis faster, you do not really need it to reach ketosis. Keto dieting alone will allow you to enter that metabolic state. The most important adjustment for a healthier lifestyle is a well-rounded low-carb diet, which is found by following the ketogenic diet.

If you have decided to take part in the two simultaneously, you should do so when you are already in a state of ketosis. This will make fasting more manageable for you to cope with as your body is already making use of fat as an energy source, and you do not need to have extra carbohydrates to fuel your system. You should also be careful with choosing the fasting method that will suit your needs and doesn't push you beyond your limits.

Tips for a Successful Keto and Fasting Plan

At this point, we figure that you have most likely decided to combine the keto diet and intermittent fasting. If you wish to go the extra mile to achieve these positive results, you can combine the two; however, as with every new health experience of this nature, you should consult your doctor before you begin. Before you start on this path, though, here are some guidelines that you should consider incorporating into your plan to achieve the best results.

1. Eat enough

Naturally, intermittent fasting ensures that you eat less during the day. Regardless of that, try to continue to eat healthy keto-friendly foods to help your system stay away from deficits and metabolic difficulties. With the help of an app or website, you can track the ideal caloric level for your body, as well as your essential macronutrients for each day. These will also help you monitor them to ensure that you are getting enough nutrients daily. It is necessary to get a sufficient amount of fats during the fasting period from either seed, olive oil, or avocado. Also, you should add protein sources, as well as some low-carb vegetables to incorporate fiber into your diet.

2. Measure your ketone levels

Although fasting will help you stay in ketosis for a more extended period, make sure that you are not eating too many carbs or anything capable of jolting you out of ketosis. It is imperative for you to keep track of your ketone level to guarantee that you are always in this metabolic state.

3. Start with shorter fasting windows

If you are combining a keto diet and intermittent fasting, the best way to go about it is, to start off with short fasting windows. This allows you to then build them up as you get used to the practice and make it into a routine. Using the keto diet as a base is one of the most widely practiced strategies out there. With the keto diet as a guide, you can also do the 24-hour fast and eat a ketogenic meal once a day. Adding the 16:8 fasting method to your plan is also an excellent decision. You fast for 16 hours in a day and only consume your keto-friendly meals during the eight-hour window.

4. Plan your meals

The focal point of the keto diet is the need to eat the proper amount of fats daily. Intermittent fasting, on the other hand, focuses on the reduction of the number of times you eat every day. Combining both practices consist of you putting in extra effort by paying more attention to not just what you eat but how you eat as well. The ideal approach is to plan your meals and snacks more than you did ordinarily.

5. Know the facts

When you are combining two different plans, it is vital to keep a few points in mind to help you determine if you should continue with it and ensure that you will achieve success.

    a. Restrictive dietary patterns do not lead to weight loss.

If you are thinking of ways to maintain a healthy lifestyle, you should first consider the possibility of avoiding processed foods, reducing the intake of calories, and cutting added sugar and carbohydrate sources like bread, pasta, baked goods, and so on. You should also increase your physical activities. For someone who wants to lose weight, it is not necessary to follow a restrictive dietary pattern. Try other opportunities and keep the restrictive nutritional habits such as intermittent fasting and keto diet as your last resort.

    b. Intermittent fasting and the keto diet are not recommended for everyone.

We have said this numerous times because it is important. Although the practice of combining intermittent fasting and the keto diet is relatively safe for most people, it is not recommended for everybody. Therefore, before you get started with both programs, make sure that it will not be detrimental to your health by figuring out if you belong to a group of people for whom the diet is applicable for.

    c.   There are no conclusive reports to support both plans yet.

For what it's worth, the combination of the keto diet and intermittent fasting does not have strong scientific backings yet. Summer Yule, a registered dietician, once said that she will not recommend the combo because there is no research on humans that speak of its benefits.

6. Do not become overwhelmed

Jumping into the keto diet and intermittent fasting may be overwhelming and too much for you to handle. To avoid feeling like that, you should either begin with one before trying the other or vice versa. This way, your body should have adjusted to one before experimenting by adding the other.

Tips on Getting Comfortable With Intermittent Fasting

We thought that it would be significant to give you specific suggestions if you decide to try out intermittent fasting. Fasting can be tedious for some people, and we aim to help you ease into it gradually.

- Water is critical whenever you are fasting, even in days when you will be eating. Be sure to drink at least 8 glasses of water per day.
- It is vital to stay busy while on your fast. Being idle will cause the program to weigh heavily on you and may tempt you to give up.
- Whenever you decide to fast, make sure that critical tasks are done before the early hours of the day. A night before your fast, plan your day and work on a to-do list (if possible). Besides, all important tasks should be done in the hours after breakfast to keep your mind occupied.
- To see a noticeable result with your efforts, you need to give yourself time. Wait for at least three weeks before deciding if your aim is yielding anything tangible or not. Stay on the program consistently in that period as well to be able to come to a conclusion.

- As you proceed with the fast, monitor your progress. The best way to do this is by taking pictures. When you associate yourself with the progress that you are making, then it will be easier to decide if your body is changing for the better or not. It is not just about the scale alone, but how you feel.
- Before starting either keto dieting or intermittent fasting, the involvement of your doctor is vital. He or she is in the best position to decide if it is beneficial for you.
- For people who want to attempt intermittent fasting, the best approach is to grow into it.

You can do this by delaying breakfast gradually, depending on the type of fats you are going for. You can shift your first meal to either 11 A.M. or noon.
- As soon as you get out of bed every day, drink a glass of water. We recommend adding mint leaves or sliced lemon to it. This will give the extra beverage flavor and make it quite nutritious.
- If you wish to try the alternate-day fasting, we recommend that you limit this to two times a week. Going for more days than that will just force your body to function too hard.
- It is essential to stick to healthy meals only. Choose the recommended keto meal plans that we have analyzed in the earlier part of this book, as a guide. Also, eat more fruits and vegetables when you are not fasting.
- Be sure not to live a boring life due to this lifestyle. Go out and have fun; don't pass on a night out with your girlfriends or buddies in the name of fasting. Nevertheless, you should watch what you eat.
- Avoid junk, fast, and processed foods at all costs. These are not healthy and will cancel out the expected results you aim for.
- Motivate yourself by having visual reminders of why you are doing this, e.g., stickers with messages in strategic places of the house. This way, you get to stay on track and keep inspired to continue. These are great, especially when a hunger pang comes at you with everything in

its arsenal.
- We need you to understand that breakfast is not the most important meal of the day. Your first meal is. So, make it delicious, nutritious, healthy, and keto-friendly.

Though intermittent fasting may seem uncomfortable at the beginning, keep going and don't give up on it. Give yourself enough time to adjust, your body will get used to fasting, and you will soon discover you no longer feel as hungry between feeding periods as you used to be. While fasting does not necessarily have to be a part of the ketogenic diet, it is absolutely possible to combine the two. If you wish to get the best out of them, it is essential for you to put in some effort to use them in the best ways possible.

Some Avoidable Mistakes

When you are on a keto diet, it is vital to keep in mind that the elimination of carbs for a high-fat diet is not a permanent change. Even though there is no adequate research to support the dangers of staying on a keto diet for a very long time, suggestions are pointing to the fact that continuing on ketosis for months on end may result in kidney stones, liver problems, osteoporosis, and high cholesterol. This is the reason why most experts advise people to remain on a keto diet for only three to six months at the most and then reintroduce carbs on certain days in specific intervals.

As for fasting, you should realize that you do not have to fast every day to procure all its benefits. As a matter of fact, subjecting yourself to fasting daily will make you weak, fatigued, and irritable. The focus should be on eating ketogenic meals first before you add fasting to your routine later. Being flexible will help you sustain the keto diet and intermittent fasting lifestyle for a more extended period.

On a final note, you should not make the mistake of ignoring those subtle or apparent signals that are sent by your body. If you are having some issues, consider increasing your carbohydrate and caloric intake a little bit. You can reduce the number of your fasting days every week as well. If that still is not helping and you feel sluggish, fatigued, or weak at any point, make sure to consult your physician, again, before continuing on with the programs.

Conclusion

Now that we have come to the end of this fantastic journey, we really do hope that you have enjoyed every bit of this ride as much as we have. At this point, we believe that you are fully equipped and for your own weight-loss journey while setting your sights on all the other health benefits that come with the two methods that have been discussed in this book.

If you have chosen to make use of the ketogenic diet as your guide for losing weight, pay attention to our tips and tricks so that you will not find yourself running into more trouble than you bargained for. While there are a lot of perks that come with this program, there are also possible dangers that might threaten your health in the long run if proper care is not taken from the onset, as it boosts your chances of developing kidney stones, among other things.

You also need to keep in mind that it is not always easy to carry on with the diet for a long time after you have reached ketosis. Even if you have the willpower to do so, it is not advisable for you to be on the keto diet forever. It is also important to note that while you are advised to go on a high-fat diet during your ketogenic dieting period, there are good and bad fats that you are now aware of and you know how to avoid consuming those unhealthy sources of fat.

Intermittent fasting is another dependable weight-loss technique that can help you reach ketosis and lose weight. Most people have found that it is an easy way to maintain this metabolic process, and they combine it with a ketogenic diet to get better results. While there are experts who are all for the combination of these two strategies, others are not totally convinced about the need for this union and refuse to recommend it. These are some of the reasons why they are still continuing to conduct research on this. Even now, there is no conclusive study to back the claims of the propagators of the combination theory. It is, therefore, strongly advised that you should consult your doctor before you adopt any of the two methods mentioned above.

We hope that you will be able to make the best out of all this material as you continue to pursue a healthy and happy lifestyle. Good luck!

If you enjoyed this book or received value from it in any way, then I'd like to ask you for a favor: would you be kind enough to leave a review for this book on Audible? It'd be greatly appreciated!

References

Axe, J. (2018). Should you pair keto with intermittent fasting? Retrieved from https://whatsgood.vitaminshoppe.com/keto-intermittent-fasting/

Better Health Channel. (n.d.). Heart disease and food. Retrieved from https://www.betterhealth.vic.gov.au/health/conditionsandtreatments/heart-disease-and-food

BMJ. (2016). High intake of saturated fats is linked to increased risk of heart disease. Retrieved from https://www.bmj.com/content/355/bmj.i6347

Bonassa, A., and Carpinelli, A. (2018). Intermittent fasting for three months decreases pancreatic islet mass and increases insulin resistance in Wistar rats. E*ndocrine Abstracts.* 56, 519. doi: 10.1530/endoabs.56.P519

Butler, N., (2017). Can fat be good for you? Retrieved from https://www.medicalnewstoday.com/articles/141442.php

Butler, N., (2019). How to begin intermittent fasting? Retrieved from https://www.medicalnewstoday.com/articles/324882

.php

Coyle, D., (2018). Intermittent fasting for women: A beginner's guide. Retrieved from https://www.healthline.com/nutrition/intermittent-fasting-for-women

D'Andrea Meira, I., et al. (2019). Ketogenic diet and epilepsy: What we know so far. *Frontiers in Neuroscience*. doi: 10.3389/fnins.2019.00005

Designed for disease: the link between local food environments and obesity and diabetes. http://www.policylink.org/sites/default/files/DESIGNEDFORDISEASE_FINAL.PDF

Diet Doc. (n.d.). What is the origin of the ketogenic diet? Retrieved from https://www.dietdoc.com/diet-tips/ketogenic-diet-origin/

Diet review: Ketogenic diet for weight loss. (n.d.). Retrieved from https://www.hsph.harvard.edu/nutritionsource/healthy-weight/diet-reviews/ketogenic-diet/

Eenfeldt, A., (2018). The keto flu, other keto side effects, and how to cure them. Retrieved from https://www.dietdoctor.com/low-carb/keto/flu-side-effects

Eenfeldt, A., (2019). Low-carb and keto side effects & how to cure them. Retrieved from https://www.dietdoctor.com/low-carb/side-effects#badbreath

Fung, J., (2019). Intermittent fasting for beginners. Retrieved from https://www.dietdoctor.com/intermittent-fasting

Gustin, A., (2018). Intermittent fasting and ket: Can you do them both? Retrieved from https://perfectketo.com/intermittent-fasting-and-keto/

Hardick, B., (2015). An intermittent fasting guide for men & women. Retrieved from https://www.drhardick.com/intermittent-fasting-men-vs-women

Harvard Health Publishing. (n.d.). Should you try the keto diet? Retrieved from https://www.health.harvard.edu/staying-healthy/should-you-try-the-keto-diet

Harvard Health Publishing. (2015). The truth about fats: The good, the bad, and the in-between. Retrieved from https://www.health.harvard.edu/staying-healthy/the-truth-about-fats-bad-and-good

Hazmic, H. (n.d.). Intermittent fasting on keto: how does it work? Retrieved from https://www.kissmyketo.com/blogs/foods-nutrition/intermittent-fasting-on-keto-how-does-it-work

Jhaveri, A., (2017). 19 keto lunches that will help you stick to your resolutions. Retrieved from: https://greatist.com/eat/keto-lunches-that-will-help-you-stick-to-your-resolutions

Kubala, J., (2018). A keto diet meal plan and menu that can transform your body. Retrieved from https://www.healthline.com/nutrition/keto-diet-meal-plan-and-menu#meal-plan

Kubala, J., (2018). Intermittent fasting and keto: Should you combine the two? Retrieved from https://www.healthline.com/nutrition/intermittent-fasting-and-keto

Kubala, J., (2018). The keto flu: Symptoms and how to get rid of it. Retrieved from https://www.healthline.com/nutrition/keto-flu-symptoms#how-long-it-lasts

Leiva, C., (2018). How to do the keto and intermittent fasting at the same time, according to experts. Retrieved from https://www.thisisinsider.com/keto-and-intermittent-fasting-same-time-2018-10

Lindberg, R., (2018). How to exercise safely during intermittent fasting. Retrieved from https://www.healthline.com/health/how-to-exercise-safely-intermittent-fasting#2

Madell, R., and Nall, R. (2018). Good fats, bad fats, and heart disease. Retrieved from https://www.healthline.com/health/heart-disease/good-fats-vs-bad-fats#polyunsaturated-fat

Mawer, R., (2018). The ketogenic diet: A detailed beginner's guide to keto. Retrieved from https://www.healthline.com/nutrition/ketogenic-diet-101#types

McNew, A. (n.d.). 51 keto breakfast recipes to help you burn fat. Retrieved from https://blog.paleohacks.com/keto-breakfast-recipes/#

Michaeli, D., (2017). What science has to say about intermittent fasting. Retrieved from https://thedoctorweighsin.com/what-science-has-to-say-about-intermittent-fasting/

Moodie, A. (n.d.). The incredible benefits of intermittent fasting. Retrieved from https://blog.bulletproof.com/intermittent-fasting-benefits/

Nessler, T., (2009). Water and Your Diet: Staying Slim and Regular With H2O. Retrieved from https://www.webmd.com/diet/features/water-for-weight-loss-diet#1

Occhipinti, M., (2018). What is the history and evolution of the keto diet? Retrieved from https://www.afpafitness.com/blog/what-is-the-history-and-evolution-of-the-keto-diet

Olsen, N., (2018). What are the benefits of intermittent fasting? Retrieved from https://www.medicalnewstoday.com/articles/323605.php

Perfect Keto. (n.d.). Calculate your keto macros in

minutes. Retrieved from https://perfectketo.com/keto-macro-calculator/

Pinkerton, J., (2018). Tips for a successful keto diet. Retrieved from https://www.wellhappyandkind.com/blog/2017/12/18/tips-for-a-successful-keto-diet

Ruled.me (n.d.). The 10 best tips for keto diet success. Retrieved from https://www.ruled.me/the-10-best-tips-for-keto-diet-success/

Siim Land. (2018). Ketogenic fasting mimicking diet how to. Retrieved from https://siimland.com/ketogenic-fasting-mimicking-diet-how-to/

Thorpe, M., (2017). 10 solid reasons why yo-yo dieting is bad for you. Retrieved from https://www.healthline.com/nutrition/yo-yo-dieting#section11

Thrive/Strive. (n.d.). Keto dinners: 16 delicious low carb dinners to prepare tonight. Retrieved from https://thrivestrive.com/keto-dinner-ideas/

Wikipedia. (2019). Keytones. Retrieved from https://en.wikipedia.org/wiki/Ketone

Made in the USA
Middletown, DE
28 November 2019